POLYVGAL THERAPY AND VAGUS NERVE:

THE DAILY VAGUS NERVE EXERCISES TO CONTROL ANXIETY, BEAT DEPRESSION, OVERCOME TRAUMA, REDUCE THE CHRONIC ILLNESS AND ACTIVATE YOUR EMOTIONAL INTELLIGENCE.

By: James Paul Docter.

© Copyright 2020 by James Paul Docter.

All rights reserved.

All rights reserved. No part of this guide may be reproduced in any form without permission in writing from the publisher except in the case of brief quotations embodied in critical articles or reviews.

Legal & Disclaimer

The information contained in this book and its contents is not designed to replace or take the place of any form of medical or professional advice; and is not meant to replace the need for independent medical, financial, legal or other professional advice or services, as may be required. The content and information in this book has been provided for educational and entertainment purposes only.

The content and information contained in this book has been compiled from sources deemed reliable, and it is accurate to the best of the Author's knowledge, information and belief. However, the Author cannot guarantee its accuracy and validity and cannot be held liable for any errors and/or omissions. Further, changes are periodically made to this book as and when needed. Where appropriate and/or necessary, you must consult a professional (including but not limited to your doctor, attorney, financial advisor or such other professional advisor) before using any of the suggested remedies, techniques, or information in this book.

Upon using the contents and information contained in this book, you agree to hold harmless the Author from and against any damages, costs, and expenses, including any legal fees potentially resulting from the application of any of the information provided by this book. This disclaimer applies to any loss, damages or injury caused by the use and application, whether directly or indirectly, of any advice or information presented, whether for breach of contract, tort, negligence, personal injury, criminal intent, or under any other cause of action.

You agree to accept all risks of using the information presented inside this book.

You agree that by continuing to read this book, where appropriate and/or necessary, you shall consult a professional (including but not limited to your doctor, attorney, or financial advisor or such other advisor as needed) before using any of the suggested remedies, techniques, or information in this book.

CONTENTS

Chapter One: The Polyvagal Theory 1

Chapter Two: An Intro To Vagus Nerve. 27

Chapter Three: How To Stimulate The Vagus Nerve To Relieve Stress And Improve The Functioning Of The Body 63

Chapter Four: Relevance Of Vagus Nerve Stimulation 66

Chapter Five: How To Overcome A Trauma 95

Chapter Six: Chiropractic Action 100

Chapter Seven: Vagus Nerve And Anxiety: Exercises To Tone And Reduce Stress... 108

CHAPTER ONE.
THE POLYVAGAL THEORY

The Polyvagal theory is called to be one of the great revolutions in the evidence of the mind-body connection. What long-time therapists and body facilitators had been defending from an experiential or intuitive place, such as the direct connection between body and mind and the psychosomatic influence of mental and bodily experiences with each other, is now neuroscientific evidence and with extraordinary possibilities of intervention both from medicine and from therapy or personal development.

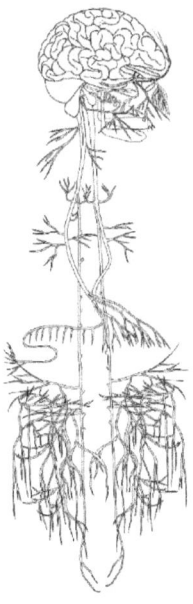

The Autonomous Nervous System regulates those vital functions that our body performs without our conscious intervention. The endocrine system, the beating of the heart and the pumping of the blood in our organism, the breathing when we do not act directly on it, are some of the examples of a multitude of actions that take place in us without our conscious direction.

The Autonomous Nervous System, or SNA, is composed of two systems with opposing activities. The sympathetic system and the parasympathetic system. Both systems regulate very different activities in the body, heart, tears, sweat, saliva, kidney behavior, intestine, sexual organs, bladder, pancreas, etc. This regulation is related to the maintenance of balance or homeostasis between the organism and the environment.

Thus the SNA increases or reduces the activity of these described organs and many others, depending on the overall somatic evaluation that the system makes of the risk or the existence of danger or threat in the environment.

The sympathetic SNA is responsible for activating the system and increasing the level of alertness; we could say and, therefore, more connected with the concept of defense or attack. And the parasympathetic is oriented to the attitude of calm and relaxation and more connected with the state of openness and encounter or emotional contact with the outside or others.

With each interaction or relational experience we have with the environment, our SNA learns and incorporates new adaptive evaluation data in potentially stressful situations. We are constantly balancing between connection or opening situations with reduced SNA activation, less intervention of the sympathetic system and more of the parasympathetic system, or situations evaluated as threatening with greater activation of the SNA through the sympathetic system.

Therefore, the SNA can say that it decisively influences our way of relating to the world and of evaluating our approach or connection with others or the experience of feeling safe and secure. And it does below the level of consciousness.

«Flight or attack are reactions governed by the sympathetic system. And they maintain a high level of activation in the body. These types of reactions are not universal but are a response to a subjective map resulting from experience, adaptive learning by the system from the experiences of past interactions.«

What does the Polyvagal Theory say, and why is it a revolution in the intervention of aid in the development of people?

Stephen Porges, an expert in the study and operation of the SNA, disseminated this theory in 1995. It shows the hierarchy system and priorities of operation of the vagal system or system regulated by the vagus nerve.

The Vago nerve is the tenth cranial nerve and connects the brain with numerous internal organs reaching the colon and has a transcendental role in the ANS directly intervening in the reduction of the activation of the sympathetic system in cases of evaluation of low risk or impossibility of defending.

The ANS basically has three types of reactions to external situations by virtue of its threat level.

Escape or attack are reactions governed by the sympathetic system. And they maintain a high level of activation in the body. These types of reactions are not universal but are a response to a subjective map resulting from experience, adaptive learning by the system based on the experiences of past interactions.

Paralysis in the face of a threat is a direct intervention by the unmyelinated vagus nerve or older part of the nerve. It is an unconscious system that starts when it is considered that there is no defense or escapes possible. It is common to all vertebrates.

Finally, there is the approach or connection strategy, the search for social interaction. This attitude also depends on a direct intervention of the vagus nerve in its most evolved part, which is the myelinated branch. His intervention reduces the activation of the defense system of the sympathetic system and regulates actions such as voice, facial expressions, and the ability to listen.

The Polyvagal theory tells us about the map of hierarchies in the role of the vagus nerve in the ANS and the relationship between the functioning of this nerve, the map of past experiences that determine its intervention, and the result in the actions of these possible three responses to the environment.

We can understand then that a trauma or constant stressful experiences in the past and especially in certain moments of life with greater load, such as childhood, can cause alterations in the scheme of evaluation of threats of the environment that remain anchored in our body in an unconscious plane and that can determine our way of relating to the world and ultimately our ability to develop as full people.

The polyvagal theory thus marks a milestone in the way of approaching now the strategies of help, therapeutic or personal development oriented through the body. From being mostly considered as collateral to acquire the focus of interventions that can be direct in many cases.

Studies on touch in 2009 have resulted in it being known that through massage or touch, depending on the lightness or the greater pressure of the massage, the sympathetic system or its reduction can be encouraged more or less through activation of vagal activity. Thus a light massage in certain areas activates the sympathetic system, and a moderate pressure massage increases the vagal activity.

"Touch stimulates the autonomic nervous system, and vagal stimulation promotes the reduction of depression, pain, and stress and increases immune function" (Diego and Field 2009)

The weight of the possible modification of the evaluation of the environment through a body intervention now acquires much greater relevance.

We hope that this neuroscientific advancement is the first of many others that are giving biological support to what, experientially, we have proven day by day those who seek to integrate body tools in our practice of human development.

Vagal paradox: the origin of polyvagal theory

The polyvagal theory emerged from an observed paradox while studying heart rate patterns in fetuses and human newborns. Bradycardia in obstetrics and neonatology is a clinical risk index and is assumed to be mediated by the vagus. In this same population, heart rate variability, or variation of time between beat and beat, is also considered a clinical index of adaptation mediated by the vagus. If the vagal cardiac tone is a positive health indicator of a fetus or a newborn when they are monitored and show heart rate variability, then how can the vagal tone be a negative health indicator when it manifests as bradycardia? Research in animals showed that both signs could be altered by sectioning the pathways of the vagus into the heart or by pharmacological blockade (that is, with atropine) interfering with the inhibitory action of the vagus on the sinoatrial node.

The resolution of this paradox derived from the observation that, through the evolution of the vertebrate autonomic nervous system, mammals developed two vagal efferent pathways: one has a respiratory rhythm, is exclusive to mammals, is myelinated, originates in an area of the brain stem known as the "ambiguous nucleus," it travels mainly to the organs located above the diaphragm and interacts with the structures of the brain stem that regulate the striated muscles of the head and face; the other has no respiratory rate, is observed in virtually all vertebrates, is not myelinated, travels primarily to the organs below the diaphragm and originates in the dorsal nucleus of the brain stem vagus.

Respiratory sinus arrhythmia: an index of cardiac vagal tone

To explore the differences between bradycardia and heart rate variability mediated by the vagus, we need to understand the neural components that mediate both responses. The mechanism that produces massive bradycardia is well known since it derives from a vagal inhibition of the sinoatrial node and can be mimicked by direct or indirect electrical stimulation of the brainstem areas. Validation experiments using similar protocols are unable to distinguish between basal tonic vagal activity and vagal activity due to acute stimulation. And stimulation studies are also not able to selectively differentiate between myelinated and non-myelinated vagal pathways. In addition, the manipulation of acute changes in a vagal efferent activity does not allow us to perceive the mechanisms that produce tonic variations in heart rate variability.

In healthy mammals, the heart does not beat with a constant frequency. Although the intrinsic discharge frequency of the sinoatrial node, the cardiac pacemaker, can be relatively fixed, it is modulated by transient inhibition of the pacemaker by the vagal pathways. When spontaneous respiratory rate manifests in the heart rate pattern, it is called respiratory sinus arrhythmia (ASR).

References to ASR emerged in the early 1900s. The functional relationship between the amplitude of the ASR and the cardiac vagal tone. He said that breathing was a functional test of the vagal control of the heart. Hering said: "It is known that a demonstrable reduction in heart rate with breathing is indicative of the function of the bums." Contemporary neurophysiology confirms these initial communications. Since the neural mechanisms that mediate ASR are well known as functional impulses of myelinated efferent vagal pathways, our research has focused on ASR and not on other measures of heart rate variability, whose origin has already been clearly defined...

The polyvagal theory: phylogenetic changes in the autonomic nervous system of vertebrates

Tracing the evolutionary changes invertebrates

rados, a phylogenetic model arises by which in mammals, two vagal pathways to the heart were developed. This pattern could be described in terms of three evolutionary phases during which the neural circuits to regulate the heart were developed. During the first phase, vertebrates were based on an unmyelinated vagus nerve with efferent pathways originating in an area of the brain stem similar to the dorsal vagal complex, which contains the origin of the efferent pathways and the termination of the afferents. As they evolved, a spinal sympathetic nervous system developed. Finally, with the appearance of mammals, there was a transition in the regulation of the autonomic nervous system. During this transition, some of the cells of origin of the vagus migrated from the dorsal nucleus of the vagus to the ambiguous nucleus. In this evolutionary process, many of the efferent vagal fibers originated in the ambiguous nucleus were myelinated and integrated into the function of brainstem regulation of the special visceral efferent pathways that regulated the striated muscles of the head and face. It is interesting that Langley established the hypothesis of a phylogenetic development of vagal fibers congruent with this description of polyvagal theory :

The hypothesis that I would point out as the approximate cause of the existence of two types of nerve fibers is that the cells with non-medulled [non-myelinated] fibers were the first in phylogeny to migrate from the central nervous system, with subsequent migration occurring when produced a subsequent specialization of the central nerve cells, and that these migrated cells gave rise to spinal [myelinated] fibers. According to this hypothesis, the two forms of embryonic cells would have persisted to a varying degree in the different vertebrates, each of them giving rise to their own type of axon.

In mammals, the unmyelinated vagal pathways that originate in the dorsal nucleus of the vagus regulate mainly the organs located below the diaphragm, although some of them end in the sinoatrial node. According to the hypothesis of polyvagal theory, these non-myelinated fibers remain fundamentally inactive until there is a vital threat, and they are probably enhanced during hypoxia and the states in which the influence of vagal impulses myelinated to the heart is depressed. This sequence can be observed, in the human fetal heart rate, in which bradycardia is more likely to appear when the tonic influence of myelinated pathways, which is manifested in ASR, is low.

In the first vertebrates, the unmyelinated vagal pathway that originated in the brain stem was a critical component of neural regulation of all viscera. This bidirectional system reduced metabolic expenditure when resources were low, as in the case of oxygen reduction. The nervous system of primitive vertebrates did not need much oxygen to survive and could decrease heart rate and metabolic demands when oxygen concentrations fell. Therefore, this circuit provided a conservation system that was adapted as a primitive defense in mammals, manifesting itself as feigned death and syncope and dissociation responses caused by trauma. Since this defense system could be deadly for mammals in demand for oxygen, it worked as a last option for survival. Non-myelinated, phylogenetically primitive vagal motorways are shared with most vertebrates, and, in mammals, when not recruited as a defense system, they function as support for health, growth, and repair through regulation via Neural subdiaphragmatic organs (i.e., internal organs that are located below the diaphragm).

The myelinated vagal circuit with efferents originating in the brainstem called "ambiguous nucleus" is exclusive to mammals. The "newer" myelinated vagal motorways regulate the supradiaphragmatic organs (e.g., the heart and lungs) and integrate into the brain stem with structures that modulate the striated muscles of the head and face through special visceral efferent pathways, leading to a system of functional social interaction. This newer vagal circuit slows the heart rate and maintains calm states.

POLYVAGAL THEORY: THE EMERGENCE OF THE SOCIAL INTERACTION SYSTEM

The integration of myelinated vagal cardiac pathways with the neural regulation of the face and head gave rise to the system of social interaction of mammals. As illustrated in Figure 29-1, the nerve impulses of the social interaction system consist of a somatomotor component and a visceromotor component. The somatomotor component consists of the visceral efferent pathways that regulate the striated muscles of the head and face. The visceromotor component is formed by the myelinated supradiaphragmatic vagus, which regulates the heart and bronchi. Functionally, the social interaction system originates from a cardiofacial connection, which coordinates the heart with the muscles of the face and head. The initial function of the system is to coordinate suction-swallowing-breathing-vocalization. Atypical coordination of this system in the early stages of life is indicative of subsequent difficulties in social behavior and emotional regulation.

When we have a complete interaction, two important biobehavioral characteristics of this system are expressed. First, body status is regulated effectively to promote growth and repair (e.g., visceral homeostasis). This is done functionally through an increase in the influence of the myelinated vagal motor pathways on the cardiac pacemaker to slow the heart rate, inhibit the fight or flight mechanisms of the sympathetic nervous system, attenuate the stress response system of the hypothalamic axis. Pituitary-adrenal (HHS; responsible for cortisol release) and reduce inflammation by modulating immune reactions (e.g., cytokines). Second, the cardiofacial phylogenetic connection of mammals intervenes by transmitting the physiological state through facial expression and prosody (voice intonation), as well as regulating the muscles of the middle ear to modulate the frequency of listening

The nuclei of origin of the brain stem of the social interaction system are influenced by higher brain structures (i.e., top-down impulses) and visceral afferents (i.e., bottom-up impulses). The direct corticobulbar pathways reflect the influence of the frontal areas of the cortex (that is, upper motor neurons) on the bulbar nuclei of the origin of this system. Bottom-up influences take place through feedback by the afferent vagus (e.g., solitary tract), transmitting information from the visceral organs to the bulbar nuclei (e.g., nucleus of the solitary tract) and influencing both in the nuclei of origin of the system as in the prosencephalic areas that are supposed to be involved in several psychiatric disorders. In addition, the anatomical structures involved in social interaction have a neurophysiological relationship with the HHS axis, social neuropeptides (peg, oxytocin, and vasopressin), and the immune system.

The afferents of the target organs of the social interaction system, including the muscles of the face and head, also provide powerful afferent impulses to the nuclei of origin, regulating the visceral and somatic components of the system. The nucleus of origin of the facial nerve forms the limit of the ambiguous nucleus, and the afferents of the trigeminal nerve provide primary sensory impulses to the ambiguous nucleus. Therefore, the anterior vagal complex, formed by the ambiguous nucleus and the trigeminal and facial nerve nuclei, is functionally related to the expression and experience of emotions. Activation of the somatomotor component (e.g., listening, ingestion or elevation of the eyelids) could trigger visceral changes that would support social interaction while modulating the visceral state, depending on whether there is an increase or decrease in the influence of the Vaginal efferents myelinated to the sinoatrial node (i.e., increase or decrease of the vagal brake), would induce or prevent such behavior. For example, the stimulation of visceral states that encourage mobilization (i.e., fight or flight behaviors) avoids the ability to express social interaction behaviors.

The cardiofacial connection allowed mammals to detect if a congener was in a state of physiological calm and if it was "safe" to approach, or if he was physiologically reactive and highly mobilized, during which time the interaction would be dangerous. At the same time, this connection allows the individual to signal "security" through patterns of facial expression and vocal intonation and potentially calm an agitated congener to establish a social relationship. When the newest mammalian bum functions optimally in social interactions (that is, it inhibits sympathetic stimulation that induces fighting or flight behaviors), emotions are well regulated, vocal prosody is rich, and the autonomic state maintains spontaneous social relationship behaviors serene. With this newer myelinated vagal circuit, the cardiofacial system is bidirectional, influencing positive social interactions, and these are the vagal function to optimize health, reduce physiological states related to stress and support recovery and growth. Social communication and the ability to regulate relationships with each other through reciprocal interaction systems lead to a sense of connection and is an important defining characteristic of human experience.

POLYVAGAL THEORY: DISSOLUTION

The human nervous system, similar to that of other mammals, was developed not only to survive in safe environments but also to promote survival in dangerous and life-threatening environments. In order to achieve this adaptive flexibility, the autonomic nervous system of mammals, in addition to the myelinated vagal pathway integrated into the social interaction system, retained two more primitive neural circuits to regulate defense strategies (i.e., fighting behaviors). Flight and pretending of death). It is important to note that social behavior and communication and visceral homeostasis are incompatible with the neurophysiological states that maintain the defense. The strategies of the polyvagal response to challenges are phylogenetically ordered, and the newest components of the autonomic nervous system response act first. This model of autonomic reactivity is consistent with John Hughlings Jackson's concept of dissolution, in which he proposes that "the superior neural dispositions inhibit (or control) the inferior ones and, therefore, when the superior ones become suddenly non-functional, the inferior ones increase inactivity. In this hierarchy of adaptive responses, the newest social interaction circuit is used first; if that circuit fails to provide security, the oldest circuits are sequentially recruited.

POLYVAGAL THEORY: NEUROCEPTION

The polyvagal theory proposes that the neural risk assessment does not require conscious knowledge or function through the nervous circuits we share with our phylogenetic vertebrate ancestors. Therefore, the term "neuroception" was introduced to emphasize a different neural process of perception, capable of distinguishing environmental (and visceral) characteristics that are safe, dangerous, or life-threatening (29, 30). In safe environments, the autonomic state is adaptively regulated to attenuate sympathetic activation and protect the oxygen-dependent central nervous system, especially the cortex, from the metabolically conservative reactions of the dorsal vagal complex (e.g., vasovagal syncope).

Neuroception was proposed as a "reflex" mechanism capable of instantly changing the physiological state. Neuroception is a plausible mechanism that mediates the expression and alteration of positive social behavior, emotional regulation, and visceral homeostasis. Neuroception could be triggered by distinctive detectors that involve areas of the temporal cortex that communicate with the central nucleus of the tonsil and the periaqueductal gray substance since limbic reactivity is modulated by the responses of the temporal cortex to biological movements as voices, faces, and hand movements. The concept of neuroception includes the ability of the nervous system to react to the "intention" of these movements. Functionally, neuroception decodes and interprets the assumed objective of the movements and sounds of living and inanimate objects. This process takes place without the intervention of consciousness. Although we are not usually aware of the stimuli that trigger the different neuroceptive responses, we are aware of the reactions of our bodies. Therefore, the neuroception of family individuals and individuals with adequately prosodic and warm voices and expressive faces translates into a positive social interaction that promotes a sense of security.

POLYVAGAL THEORY: THE AUTONOMOUS STATE IS AN INTERMEDIATE VARIABLE

The polyvagal theory proposes that the physiological state is a fundamental part, and not a correlate, of emotion and mood. According to the theory, the autonomous state functions as an intermediate variable that skews our detection and evaluation of environmental keys. Depending on the physiological state, the same keys will be reflexively evaluated as neutral, positive, or threatening. Functionally, a change of state will change access to different brain structures and will maintain social communication or defensive fight/flight or block behavior. Contemporary research on the impact of vagus nerve stimulation on cognitive function and emotional regulation supports this model. The theory emphasizes the bidirectional relationship between the brain and the viscera, which would explain how thoughts change physiology and how the physiological state influences thoughts. As individuals change their facial expression, the intonation of their voice, their breathing pattern, and their posture, they are also modifying their physiology mainly through circuits that involve the myelinated vagal pathways to the heart.

POLYVAGAL THEORY: THE ROLE OF VISCERAL AFFERENTS IN THE REGULATION OF THE HEART

The prevalent focus of research in the investigation of the neural regulation of the heart has focused on the efferent pathways that leave the nuclei of the brain stem and the sympathetic ganglia. Limited research has been conducted on the influence of visceral afferents on the neural regulation of the heart and how these influences manifest in the regulation of the heart and other visceral organs. This is due, in part, to the efferent bias of medical training, which has resulted in a limited conceptualization of the neural regulation of the heart. However, this error is changing rapidly due to vagus nerve stimulation, a bottom-up model that focuses on the vagus as an afferent nerve (approximately 80% of vagal fibers are sensitive). It is interesting that the side effects of vagus nerve stimulation are often due to the influence of the stimulation of the efferent pathways. These side effects can be seen mainly on the characteristics of the social interaction system, with voice changes and swallowing difficulties. However, in some cases, stimulation has manifested in subdiaphragmatic organs leading to diarrhea. As vagal stimulation is more frequently applied to medical disorders, there will be an emerging awareness of the action of vagal afferent impulses on neurophysiological function (e.g., epilepsy), emotional state (e.g., depression) and cognition (e.g., learning and attention).

According to the polyvagal theory, the nuclei of origin of the myelinated vagus are regulated by complex neural circuits, involving both visceral afferents (that is, from the bottom up) and higher brain structures (that is, from top to bottom) that influence the nuclei brainstem that control myelinated vagus and striated muscles of the head and face (i.e., the social interaction system). As the function of visceral afferents is incorporated into the knowledge of the autonomic nervous system, clinicians and researchers will begin to recognize the manifestations of vagal control of the heart in patients with various organ disorders.

I peripherals. Instead of the interpretation of atypical neural regulation of the heart, which may reflect some forms of heart and cardiovascular disease, concomitant diseases will be interpreted not as correlates but as manifestations of the dysfunction of a "system" consistent with Walter's prophetic vision. Hess

Several chronic diseases that manifest in specific subdiaphragmatic organs (e.g., kidney, pancreas, liver, intestine, genitals, etc.) have identifiable characteristics that have led to treatments directed at the target organs (e.g., drugs or surgery). However, other disorders that impact the quality of life, such as irritable bowel syndrome and fibromyalgia, are defined by nonspecific symptoms. The medical literature relates these nonspecific chronic diseases with atypical vagal regulation of the heart, which is reflected in a decrease in heart rate variability Congruent with these findings, frequency variability has been proposed as a biomarker of these disorders.

The polyvagal theory proposes an alternative interpretation of this covariance. In contrast, the decrease in variability is proposed as a neurophysiological marker of a diffuse readjustment of the autonomic nervous system after a complex adaptive reaction to the threat. This interpretation supports the existence of an intense connection between the prevalence of a history of abuse, especially sexual abuse in women, and the manifestations of nonspecific clinical disorders, such as irritable bowel syndrome and fibromyalgia. In addition, emotional stress intensifies the symptoms and hinders the positive outcome of the treatment, while traumas can trigger or aggravate the symptoms (37, 38). We propose that a neural response initially adaptive to the threat, through visceral afferent feedback from the organs to the brain stem, can lead to a chronic reorganization of the autonomic regulation observed in the vagal regulation of the heart (i.e., depression of heart rate variability) together with an impaired function and afferent painful signal of subdiaphragmatic organs.

Neurocardiology defines an emerging discipline that provides an opportunity to study two-way communication between the brain and the heart. Looking at living organisms as a collection of dynamic, adaptive, interactive, and interdependent physiological systems, it becomes clear that the autonomic nervous system cannot be considered functionally separated from the central nervous system. Consistent with the polyvagal theory, the heart is not "floating in a sea of viscera," but is metaphorically anchored in the central structures by efferent pathways and continuously receives regulatory signals from the central structures through abundant afferent pathways. Therefore, the treatment and assessment of cardiac function and other manifestations of autonomic dysfunction in the neural regulation of the heart should be based on the bi-directional connections between the autonomic and central brain structures. This knowledge informs us of the vulnerability of heart disease and dysfunction associated with the induction of the autonomic nervous system in chronic states of defense, as well as the adaptation that promotes functional modulation through the social interaction system.

The theory emphasizes the role of the heart in social behavior. The theory states that the vagus nerve, a nerve found only in mammals, provides information to the heart to direct behaviors as complex as establishing relationships with other people or abandoning other relationships. A distinctive aspect of the polyvagal theory is that it does not focus on the heart rate per se, but rather on the variability of the heart rate (HRV), a variable previously considered uninteresting, in the order of noise.

Since 1995, a wide range of research has emerged in support of the polyvagal theory and has demonstrated the importance of the heart in social functioning. In 2001, Porges and his colleagues measured children when they were engaged in social interaction with the experimenter (the latter cooed, talked to them and smiled at them), and when they encountered the experimenter showing them that a neutral face - a frozen expression. Not only did children's HRVs increase during social interaction, but increases in HRVs were predictive of positive engagement during this interaction (increased attention and active participation by children). In adults too, HRV seems to be associated with being able to regulate emotions during social interaction, with extraversion, and generally, with a positive mood.

Have you ever felt like a threat for no particular reason? Dr. Porges' polyvagal theory suggests that we have an unconscious sensing system that interprets the danger signs we perceive without realizing it.

There are many processes that can occur in our bodies and in our minds. And this without our being fully aware of it. The polyvagal theory tries to provide an explanation for one of these processes, which we can often regard as intuitive.

In this sense, we may have already experienced the feeling of being in danger without finding a reason to justify it. We sometimes feel threatened even if no one around us seems to be affected or embarrassed by anything in particular.

We travel the world by reading a multitude of social signals. When we interact with others, we unconsciously compile facial expressions, body movements, and tones of voice. As our brains and bodies interpret these signals, our sense of self is shaped by them and by our environment.

The information that our bodies process through these signals tells us who we can trust and who we cannot. We interpret who or what may be a danger to us, adopting one position or another as an answer.

Neuroception and polyvagal theory

Dr. Porges is the originator of the polyvagal theory, which describes the process by which neural circuits are able to decipher danger indices in our environment as neuroception. Neuroception would thus be what makes us experience the world by involuntarily exploring people and the environment to determine if they are safe or if, on the contrary, they pose some threat to us.

It is a totally unconscious process that takes place in our autonomic nervous system, in the same way, that we breathe without making any voluntary effort for it. It's an automatic detection system that looks for danger signs.

Detection in our environment

This involuntary detection in search of signals of any potential danger occurs from birth and is extremely important in our survival. Our body is designed from birth to observe, process, and respond.

Babies respond to feelings of danger, safety, or closeness to their parents and the people who care for them. It happens from birth. We spend the rest of our lives unconsciously detecting these dangers or safety signs.

The three stages of response development

According to the polyvagal theory, Porges describes three evolutionary stages involved in the process. The polyvagal theory considers the interaction between the sympathetic and parasympathetic nervous systems is not just a question of balance. Porges considers that there is a hierarchy of responses integrated into our autonomous nervous system, which takes place in 3 stages.

Immobilization: the most basic path. The immobilizing response to danger signs involves the vagus nerve, the back of which response to signs of extreme danger. This causes our parasympathetic nervous system to activate at full speed, and the bodily response will immobilize us.

Mobilization: this occurs from the sympathetic nervous system;

What is the sympathetic nervous system?

The sympathetic nervous system is one of the branches of the autonomic nervous system. We are faced with a type of structure that takes on a large number of involuntary functions. Tasks like heart rate control, digestion, sweating, etc. are dimensions regulated by the sympathetic, parasympathetic, or enteric nervous system.

The sympathetic nervous system is one that takes on a series of very concrete tasks: regulating and activating our reflexes and reactions. As we have already indicated, it is this organic center that allows us to react to any "non-neutral" emotional stimulus. This involves, for example, a stressful situation, whether mild or intense, as a study by the Welfare University in Osaka reveals to us.

It is made up of 23 nodes that start from the spinal bulb. They connect on both sides of the spinal cord and the organs they innervate.

In addition, this system is made up of two types of neurons. The first is the pre-ganglion neurons, which connect to the spinal cord and to the lymph node. To be able to carry out their functions, they need a concrete neurotransmitter: acetylcholine.

The other type of neuron found in the sympathetic system is the post-ganglion neuron. The latter needs norepinephrine to be able to connect to the ganglion and the organ it innervates (heart, liver, stomach, intestines, lungs, etc.).areas of the sympathetic system

It is important to know how the sympathetic system is structured. We have just seen how it connects: let's now see how it works.

Exit area. The sympathetic system starts, as we have pointed out, from the medulla oblongata, the nucleus which regulates a large spectrum of unconscious but vital functions.

- The sympathetic cervical area, where the entire nerve formation of the head and neck is located.
- Superior cardiac area, with all the visceral vascular branches relating to the carotid plexus, the submaxillary zone, the pharynx, the larynx, etc.
- The sympathetic thoracic area. It is a region that encompasses both sides of the spine, with joints, intercostal nerves, etc.
- Lumbar area. This includes the psoas muscle, the inferior vena cava, etc.
- The pelvic area, which goes from the sacral areas to the rectum.

What happens in your body when the sympathetic nervous system is activated?

People who suffer from daily stress will like to know what happens in their bodies during these situations. What is more, if we have something as common as hypertension, it may be important to know what role the sympathetic nervous system plays and how it affects our health. In fact, studies like the one in the Journal of Human Stress tell us how this bond is created and what the differences are between men and women in it.

How the sympathetic system works

The mechanism of action of the sympathetic system, in the event of danger or anxiety, is one of the most complex processes in existence. Now let's see how he reacts to a threatening stimulus:

It promotes the release of adrenaline and norepinephrine into the bloodstream through the kidneys. The goal is simple: we need more energy and activation to be able to react. This energy requires, for example, that the liver produces more glucose.

It increases the heart rate to bring us more oxygen and nutrients through the blood.

Bronchodilation takes place. This means that we need more oxygen and that our lungs are working as much as they can.

All activities related to digestion slow down. We cannot forget that this process requires great energy and that, in times of stress and alarm, this task is secondary. The brain just wants us to react, to face this stimulus, or to flee.

Also, and just as importantly, the sympathetic system produces mydriasis or pupillary dilation. This unconscious reaction allows us to increase our visual field and react more safely.

It's the one who helps us to mobilize in dangerous situations and thus to face a threat. Polyvagal theory suggests that this path develops as an evolutionary hierarchy.

Social commitment: this is the last acquisition that humans have developed in the hierarchy of responses. Social engagement responds to the ventral part of the lower nerve. It is the part of the nerve that responds to feelings of security and connection. Social engagement is a process that allows us to feel grounded in feelings of engagement. But also security and tranquility

The impact of the trauma

In people who have experienced trauma, especially for whom immobilization has occupied an important place in this trauma, one can observe a severe distortion of the ability to detect the environment in search of danger signs.

One of the functions of this system is that the person can no longer be in a vulnerable position. Indeed, the body will do what is necessary to avoid it. This can significantly increase sensitivity, interpreting signs that are neutral as false positives.

Many of the signs that are interpreted as harmless, even benign by other people, are read as synonymous with the threat by people who have suffered trauma. A change in facial expression, a particular tone of voice, or certain body postures can put them unconsciously in a protective posture.

The vagus nerve and polyvagal theory

Our vagus nerve is branched by many areas of our body. It has a fundamental role in the influence of the cranial nerves that regulate social engagement through facial expression and vocalization.

As humans, we yearn for feelings of security and confidence in our interactions with others. In addition, we quickly learn to interpret the signs that tell us that we are not safe. This is precisely why, as we strengthen our relationships with other people, we can more easily build healthier relationships. And experience better quality intimacy with others.

PORGES AND THE POLIVAGAL THEORY: IMPLICATIONS IN TRAUMA

Porges has developed polyvagal theory, a theory that explains how the autonomic nervous system (SNA) is involved in the regulation of viscera, social interaction, attachment, and emotions. His studies defend that the SNA is formed by two main branches, the sympathetic one that is related to the alert (sweating, redness, tension, etc.) and the parasympathetic that activates relaxation and calm, would be like the accelerator and the brake of a car. The nuance that Porges brings is that the parasympathetic branch would be divided in turn into two different branches.

Throughout evolution, we have developed two branches of this parasympathetic nerve:

Vague ventral. Evolutionarily more recent, it is myelinated. We share it with mammals. It is related to social behavior and interpersonal communication, activates the sensation of calm when the danger has passed, and regulates the cardiac tone, viscera, and facial signs when there is tranquility.

Dorsal vagus: It is phylogenetically more primitive and not myelinated. We share the reptiles and, when activated, causes immobilization.

Nature has been creating, throughout evolution, three neural systems that regulate behavioral and physiological adaptation to social situations, threats, and moments in which life is in danger. The three phylogenetic stages would be:

The sympathetic branch of the SNA. It is related to the activation of the viscera (for example, acceleration of breathing and heart rate). It is activated in fight-flight situations.

The myelinated branch of the vagus nerve. It is related to social communication. It allows immobilization without being traumatic because the person feels relaxed and calm (for example, in sexual intercourse or when sleeping). Promotes the physiological regulation of calm after the activation of the sympathetic branch.

The non-myelinated and more evolutionarily primitive branch of the vagus nerve. It is related to immobilization, dissociation, or collapse behaviors. It is activated in situations where a threat is perceived that exceed the person's resources or threatens his life. The situation of immobilization that it causes is optimal for reptiles because it helps them stay a long time without breathing and be still to regulate their temperature, but their activation is extremely traumatic for mammals

The polyvagal theory of Porges has a crucial value for psychologists because it allows us to understand why in a situation that causes a lot of stress or fear, paralysis occurs at the body level, and at the mental level, it causes traumatic dissociation of the personality and somatic dissociation. It allows us to understand how important a child's sense of safety with their caregivers or a patient with their therapist is if there is no security, effective therapy cannot be done.

When the brain perceives some danger, the amygdala is activated, which sends a signal to the body through the ANS. First, the parasympathetic branch is activated, trying not to activate the sympathetic one, which is much more expensive energy. The steps taken by the SNA in the face of danger are going in the opposite direction to the evolutionary acquisition:

Social response: The first answer would be for help. Social support is sought. In the case of babies and children, physical and emotional contact with caregivers is sought.

Mobilization fight/flight: If the aid does not appear or is not enough, a sympathetic activation occurs. Supports motor and metabolic defense activity. If this also does not resolve the perception of lack of security, then dorsovagal circuits are activated.

Immobilization: When both fight and flight are impossible, the dorsovagal branch is activated, which causes a response of immobilization and apnea (asphyxiation) with bradycardia (the heart beats slower). In adults, it is activated when it feels that life is in danger. In babies and children, it is activated when the threat is perceived as excessive, and there are no cognitive or emotional resources to face it. The lower the child's age and, therefore, the scarcer his resources, the more easily the dorsovagal branch will be activated. Immobilization is not traumatic in cases where there are emotional bonds of trust, either with caregivers at an early age or with other adults at later ages. If the immobilization is caused by someone who generates security, the ventrobasal branch that promotes emotional connection and relaxation is activated.

The activation of the dorsovagal branch seeks immobilization in mammals as a way of escaping possible predators and not wasting resources, but it is extremely traumatic in humans. A baby or child who perceives a danger that overflows their coping abilities can suffer a fear immobilization, causing a very characteristic stupor in very scared or abandoned children.

The more times there has been immobilization (or freezing) at an early age, the more likely they are to be repeated in the future. This explains why people who have suffered child abuse (psychological, physical, or sexual) tend not to react and inhibit themselves when they are abused as adults.

MISCONCEPTIONS ABOUT TRAUMA, THE INJURIES THAT COME WITH US

How to control an obsessive-compulsive disorder?

We still maintain misconceptions about trauma today. People are vulnerable, but we sometimes forget how tenacious we can be. So, as Viktor Frankl said, having an abnormal reaction to an abnormal situation is something perfectly normal, a natural response that will finally allow us to bring out our strongest / most resistant side.

Many psychologists and psychiatrists who are experts in dealing with traumatic events often remind us that all of us, at some point in our lives, will suffer from a more or less serious adverse event for which we will not be prepared. It could be the loss of a loved one, an accident, the sight of something shocking, an assault, a natural disaster, or a medical emergency.

These are situations that generate a strong impact on our brain. They stimulate the areas related to fear and the feeling of alertness, and everything soon begins to fragment around us. The prefrontal cortex, a structure that helps us to think and reason clearly, loses its strength, its agility, and our mental approach becomes more opaque, more cloudy, plunging us into a characteristic state of anxiety.

It is therefore very possible that many of our readers are aware of this experience, this situation. It is important to understand that when this happens, and always depending on the severity of this traumatic impact, our brain does not recover overnight. Or even from month to month. Healing an injured brain trapped in post-traumatic stress takes time, requires effort and adequate coping strategies.

To achieve this, it will be useful to know that there are misconceptions about trauma, which must be eliminated to initiate a more optimal, more correct approach. Let's see this below.

MISCONCEPTIONS ABOUT TRAUMA

1. Misconceptions about trauma: a traumatic event destroys our lives

When a therapist begins to work with the victim of abuse, with a person who has been assaulted, who has experienced the loss of a loved one, etc., he very often listens to the following sentence from his patient: "I will never be happy again."

It is very complicated at the beginning for this person to appreciate a fact: in reality, the trauma has a double nature. On the one hand, he has an undeniable destructive ability, but the paradox is that he also manages to transform the person to bring him back to life with greater tenacity, with better personal resources.

Suffering personally from adversity does not condemn us to eternal pain to life imprisonment. If we seek resources, support, and combine willpower and effort, the brain can be reprogrammed. The injury will not go away, but it will hurt less, and we can have a good life.

2. The trauma appears following a threatening event

If we refer to the way trauma is defined in the Diagnostic and Statistical Manual of Mental Disorders, we will see that it appears as "what happens after the experience of the death of a loved one, of a threat real, of a serious injury such as an assault, disasters, abuse or life-threatening diseases."

In reality, many nuances can be introduced into this definition. First, trauma does not appear as a "reaction" to these adverse events as such, but rather as the result of an "emotional and psychological effect" it has on the person in particular. More importantly, the same event can sometimes cause trauma in some people, not others.

What is more, when something shocking happens, the reaction is not immediate, the injury is never instantaneous. It occurs later when the person begins to wonder about his own life, his own reality, and what surrounds the two.

For example, consider a person who has just been diagnosed with cancer. Perhaps this information, as such, is sufficient, at first glance, to feel defeated and traumatized. However, for many people, the most shocking thing is not always the disease itself, but not having the support of the spouse or people who cease to be present at the most difficult times.

3. Trauma is a mental illness

Another misconception about trauma is to see or understand it exclusively as "mental illness." Indeed, it is something much deeper. Currently, many subject matter experts, such as psychologist Richard Tedeschi of the University of North Carolina, prefer to approach post-traumatic stress disorder in another way.

If trauma means "injury," then we are faced with something that is "broken." For example, when someone suffers from a fall or a blow, they can have one or more bones broken. Therefore, when someone suffers from psychological trauma, a fracture also appears a mental injury, which makes it impossible for that person to be the same as before. Someone who is traumatized is "psychologically injured," and these injuries can be moral or emotional.

4. If we are strong, we can deal with the trauma on our own

We still live in a society where we consider that the one who asks for help is weak, the one who takes medicine is crazy and that the one who is strong and can achieve everything never falls. There is some data here, however: suicide rates are alarming, and those who apparently could do it all on their own couldn't even do it with their own lives. As we said before, trauma breaks us inside, and no one, absolutely no one, can run for a long time with a broken soul, a fragmented mind, and an eroded heart.

This is undoubtedly one of the most common misconceptions about trauma: believing that time heals everything, that it is better to forget than to face, that a strong attitude makes all pain go away ... don't do it, let's avoid believing that since it leads us irreparably to a dead end.

In conclusion, trauma does not deserve to convert us into people we do not want to be. We can stop feeling trapped; we deserve life more dignified and free from those weights of the past that blur our present. Let's look for help; let's actively work on this still injured inner reality and give ourselves the opportunity to transform, heal, and live fully.

CHAPTER TWO.
AN INTRO TO VAGUS NERVE.

Vagus nerve. From the Latin Nervus vagus, also known as pneumogastric, this nerve is primarily responsible for the ability to swallow, the reflex of nausea, some flavors, and part of speech.

What is the vagus nerve?

The vagus nerve is one of the cranial nerves that is distinguished by having four nuclei and five different types of fiber. Specifically, it is the cranial nerve number X and is the most predominant neural effector of the parasympathetic nervous system, since it comprises 75% of all its nerve fibers

It is known as a "vagus" nerve to mention ramblings and detours. It is the nerve whose course is the longest of the cranial nerves; they extend and distribute widely below the level of the head.

It arises in the medulla oblongata or medulla oblongata, and advances towards the jugular foramen, passing between the glossopharyngeal and spinal accessory nerves, and is composed of two ganglia: one superior and one inferior.

Starting from the medulla oblongata and through the jugular hole, the vagus nerve descends into the thorax, passing through different nerves, veins, and arteries. Both its left and right parts extend inside the neck to the thorax; This is why he is responsible for bringing part of the parasympathetic fibers to the thoracic viscera.

The vagus nerve interacts, especially with the immune system and the central nervous system, and performs motor functions in the larynx, diaphragm, stomach, heart. It also has sensory functions in the ears, tongue, and visceral organs such as the liver.

Damage to this nerve can cause dysphagia (swallowing problems), or incomplete closure of the oropharynx and nasopharynx. On the other hand, pharmacological interventions on the vagus nerve can help control different pain, for example, those that are caused by cancer and by laryngeal tumors or intrathoracic diseases.

One of the most important cranial nerves, belonging to the parasympathetic nervous system.

The vagus nerve is number 10 of the cranial nerves. Among other things, it is responsible for transmitting information related to sensory and muscular activity, as well as anatomical functions.

Cranial nerves

The lower part of our brain is composed of a complex network of nerves that we know as "cranial nerves" or "cranial nerves." In total, there are 12; they originate directly in our brain and are distributed along different fibers through holes that are at the base of the skull towards the neck, thorax, and abdomen.

Each of these nerves is composed of fibers that fulfill different functions and that arise from a specific part of the brain (it can be in the base or in the stem). Depending on their location and the specific place from which they depart, the cranial nerves are divided into subgroups:

Connection with other nerves

As we saw before, the vagus nerve connects with different nerves; that is, it exchanges several of its fibers and functions. the nerves with which it connects are the following:

- ✓ Accessory nerve.
- ✓ Glossopharyngeal nerve
- ✓ Facial nerve.
- ✓ Hypoglossal nerve
- ✓ Sympathetic nerve
- ✓ The first two spinal nerves.

- ✓ Phrenic Nerve

Its five types of fibers and their functions

Nerve fibers, or nerves, are the extensions that connect the center of each nerve cell with the next. They transmit signals that are known as action potentials and allow us to process the stimuli.

The latter are not the only types of fibers; there are also to connect and activate effector organs, muscle fibers, or glands. According to Rea (2014), the vagus nerve has the following types of fibers.

1. Brachial motor fiber

Activates and regulates the muscles of the pharynx and larynx.

2. Sensory visceral fiber

Responsible for transmitting information from a wide variety of organs, such as the heart and lungs, the pharynx and larynx, and the highest part of the gastrointestinal tract.

3. Visceral motor fiber

It is responsible for carrying parasympathetic fibers from the smooth muscle to the respiratory tract, the heart, and the gastrointestinal tract.

4. Special sensory fiber

The vagus nerve transmits information necessary for the taste of the palate and epiglottis (the fibrous cartilage that closes the entrance of the larynx during swallowing)

5. General sensory fiber

This component allows the passage of information from parts of the ear and the dura into the posterior cranial fossa.

Vagus nerve location

It is located in the jugular hole. It is part of the twelve cranial nerves:

- ✓ Olfactory nerve
- ✓ Optic nerve
- ✓ Oculomotor nerve
- ✓ Trochlear nerve
- ✓ Trigeminal nerve
- ✓ Abducens Nerve
- ✓ Facial nerve
- ✓ Auditory nerve
- ✓ Glossopharyngeal nerve
- ✓ Vagus nerve
- ✓ Accessory nerve
- ✓ Hypoglossal nerve

It is located in the carotid sheath (vasculonervical neck pack), between the internal jugular vein (laterally) and the carotid artery (medially), located on the aponeurosis and the pre-vertebral fascicles. At the level of the root of the neck, on the right side, the nerve runs anterior to the subclavian artery and penetrates the thorax. Once inside the thorax, the right and left vagus nerves to behave differently:

Left vagus nerve. It enters the thorax between the left carotid and left subclavian arteries and, at the height of the aortic arch, emits the left recurrent laryngeal nerve. After it goes down and back, it passes in front of the pulmonary pedicle before reaching the esophagus, where it contributes to form the esophageal plexus.

Right vagus nerve. It crosses in front of the right subclavian artery, and at this point, it emits the right recurrent laryngeal nerve. Then it goes down and back, passes behind the right pulmonary pedicle before reaching the esophagus, where it also helps to form the esophageal plexus, just like its left counterpart.

Within the thorax, the vagus nerves give branches to the cardiac plexus and the pulmonary plexus. Both vagus nerves make the last part of their journey through the chest along with the esophagus, and next to it, the abdominal cavity is introduced, crossing the diaphragm through the esophageal hiatus. Once in the abdominal cavity, the left vagus nerve is distributed through the stomach, while the right vagus nerve ends in the solar plexus from where it gives branches for the abdominal viscera (stomach, intestines, kidneys, and liver).

The vagus nerve is made up of:

- ✓ Parasympathetic fibers innervate the heart, lungs, and digestive tract almost to the splenic angle of the colon.
- ✓ Special visceral motor fibers innervate striated fascicles of the larynx, pharynx, and palate.
- ✓ General visceral sensory fibers come from the mucosa of the palate, pharynx, and larynx, as well as from the heart, lungs, and digestive tract.

Special visceral sensory fibers (taste) come from the value and the epiglottis.

Somatic sensory fibers innervate the posterior part of the external auditory canal and the tympanic membrane.

The vagal nuclei located in the bulb region are distributed as motor and sensory dorsal (parasympathetic), the ambiguous nucleus (special visceral motor), and the solitary tract nucleus (visceral sensitive). Somatic sensory fibers probably connect to the trigeminal sensory nucleus. The nerve leaves the bulb outside the olive in the form of small roots and the skull through the posterior torn hole, with the inferior petrosal sinus and the medially glossopharyngeal nerve and the spinal nerve and laterally internal jugular vein. It descends through the neck and thorax to the esophageal plexus, where it joins with the nerve on the other side to form the anterior and posterior vagal trunks. Next to the base of the skull, the vagus forms the upper and lower sensory ganglia.

The vagus nerve helps regulate the heartbeat, controls muscle movement, maintains the person's breathing, and transmits a variety of chemicals throughout the body. It is responsible for keeping the digestive tract in good working order, contracting the muscles of the stomach, and intestines to help process food, sends information about what is digested and what leaves the body.

When the vagus nerve is stimulated, the response is often a reduction in heart rate or breathing. In some cases, excessive stimulation can cause someone to have what is known as a vaso-vagal response, which results in fainting or coma due to their heart rate. Selective stimulation of this nerve is also used in some medical treatments; this seems to benefit people suffering from depression and epilepsy.

The vagus nerve, also known as the pneumogastric nerve, is the tenth pair of cranial nerves involved in many functions of the body.

Anatomy of the vagus nerve

- **Mixed nerve.** The vagus nerve is composed of motor, sensitive and vegetative nerve fibers
- **Even nerve.** Two in number, the vagus nerves are located on each side of the body.
- **Innervation**. The vagus nerve is the cranial nerve that covers most of the body, from the brain to the abdomen.
- **Branches**. During its journey, the vagus nerve divides into different branches innervating numerous organs :
- ✓ **Cervical branches**. At the level of the cervical portion, the vagus nerve gives a meningeal branch, an atrial branch, pharyngeal branches, superior cardiac branches, and the superior laryngeal nerve.
- ✓ **Chest branches**. At the level of the thorax, the vagus nerve gives lower cardiac branches, bronchial branches, oesophageal branches, and the lower laryngeal nerve.

✓ **Abdominal branches.** At the level of the abdomen, the vagus nerve gives gastric branches, gastric branches, celiac branches, and renal branches.

Structure

The two pneumogastric nerves are the longest of the cranial nerves, of which they form the tenth pair and those which have the longest ramifications. They leave the skull, descend into the neck behind the carotid and jugular arteriovenous pedicle and follow the esophagus into the abdomen, where they end in numerous nerve nets for the stomach, liver and other viscera abs. Throughout this journey, these voluminous nerves emit nerve nets for neighboring organs, in particular, the recurrent nerves responsible for the motor innervation of the vocal cords. They are part of the parasympathetic autonomic nervous system (which acts on the viscera) and transport the neurotransmitters, such as acetylcholine, to the cellular receptors present on the surface of the organs. These receptors, which control a specific activity, are of two types: muscarinic receptors, activated by acetylcholine and inhibited by atropine, and nicotinic receptors, activated by acetylcholine and nicotine and inhibited by ganglioplegic (substances opposing the action of acetylcholine). The former is responsible for the contraction of the gastrointestinal muscles (activation of intestinal peristalsis, contraction of the sphincters) and the activation of digestive secretions (saliva, gastric, pancreatic and intestinal juices). Activation of nicotinic receptors causes a decrease in heart rate and blood pressure, but also intestinal and bladder spasms.

Pathology

The overactivity of the pneumogastric nerves leads to an increase in gastric secretion. Certain gastric or duodenal ulcers, rebellious to medical treatment or with complications, are treated by vagotomy (surgical procedure consisting of cutting the fibers of the pneumogastric nerves)

Role and functions of the vagus nerve

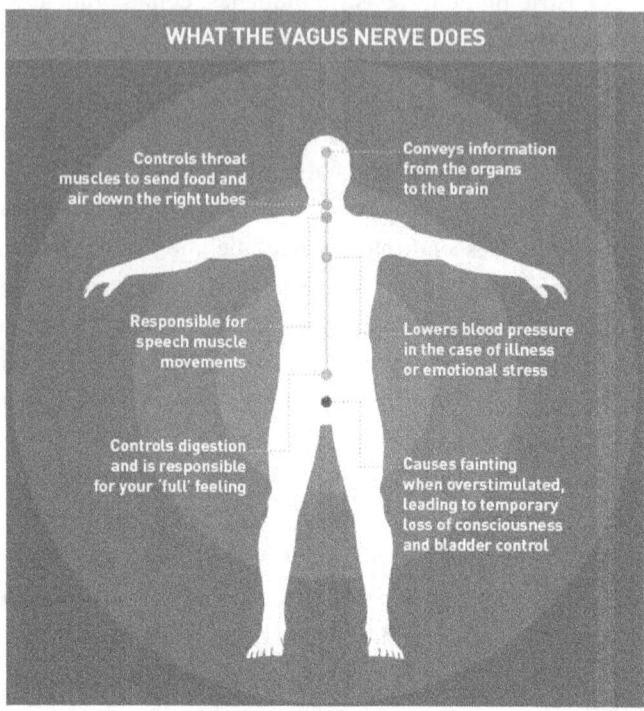

The motor, sensitive, and vegetative fibers of the pneumogastric nerve play a role in many vital functions of the organism and, in particular, the heart rate and digestive secretions.

The pneumogastric nerve is the motor for the soft palate and the pharynx. It is sensitive for the larynx, pharynx, epiglottis, soft palate, and base of the tongue. It also plays a role that is described as autonomous through the secretion of acetylcholine. The stimulation of the pneumogastric nerve, in fact, leads to the secretion of this chemical substance, which plays a role of mediator between the neurons (neuromediator). Acetylcholine slows the frequency of heartbeat, decreases the caliber of the bronchi, strengthens the contraction of the smooth muscles of the digestive tract, and increases the secretion of saliva and digestive juices.

A lesion of the pneumogastric nerve can result in a drop in the heart rate (bradycardia), a tendency to syncope and anxiety, a decrease in the caliber of the pupils (miosis), excessive sweating of the limbs, increased secretion of saliva, muscle spasms, episodes of diarrhea or breathing problems, or vagal discomfort.

HOW TO ACTIVATE THE VAGUS NERVE NATURALLY

The vagus nerve is one of twelve pairs of nerves found in the body. It is the tenth cranial nerve known to be one of the most interesting to study. Indeed, this nerve is a driving force and an internal channel that regulates fatigue and deactivates the anxious responses of our body. It is, therefore, important to know how to activate it by several practices in order to make the most of the benefits it can offer us. Let's discover together in this article some effective methods to activate the vagus nerve naturally.

VAGUS NERVE ACTIVATION, WHY IS IT SO IMPORTANT

Many situations put us in states of anxiety, fear, inconvenience, or even repulsion every day. When this happens, it is not only our moral health that is affected. One can also suffer from ailments like:

- stomach or stomach pain
- spasms
- Cramps
- agitation
- excessive and unwarranted anger

You should know that these sensations and these various ailments are instantly recovered and then amplified by the vagus nerve which sends a resounding message to the brain of the kind:

- we detect a threat

In addition, Professor Wolfgang Langhans of ETH Zurich and his team discovered a few years ago that this structure of our body is intimately linked to our emotions and concretely, with the feeling of fear or the need to escape.

Stimulating the vagus nerve, therefore, makes it possible to guard against these inconveniences and, at the same time, to permanently keep feelings of well-being.

Methods and techniques for vagus nerve activation

You should first know that activation of the vagus nerve can be performed with the help of a specialized physiotherapist through a series of massages on various parts of the body.

Here are some other methods you can use:

- breathe slowly and rhythmically into the diaphragm: by breathing from the diaphragm rather than conventionally (superficially from the top of the lungs), you can activate and tone your vagus nerve
- use an electro-activator: electro-activators make it possible to activate the desired nerve precisely. You can get it at https://www.electroactivateur.ch/128-activation-du-nerf-vague-par-electroactivation
- hum: when you hum, the vagus nerve connects to the vocal cords and is mechanically activated.
- Washing the face with cold water: a technique that is very little known, it is nonetheless effective. The repeated passage of cold water on your face activates the vagus nerve
- practice yoga
- sleep on the left side
- laugh frequently
- practice aerobic exercises
- consume foods that have a healthy intestinal flora.

Cultivating emotions, as well as simple and positive situations, allows the vagus nerve to do well. At the same time, it helps maintain good health! Such simple actions like smiling regularly, walking, or dancing can have a big positive impact on how the vagus nerve works.

Pathologies of the vagus nerve

Given the length of the vagus nerve and the various innervated organs, damage to this nerve can result in various effects, including:

- Bradycardia. It corresponds to a slowing of the heart rate. This cardiac arrhythmia may be due to the activity of the vagus nerve.
- Vagal syncope. Also called vagal discomfort: What is vagal discomfort? Vagal discomfort, also known as "syncope," results in loss of consciousness for a few seconds. It is due to the sudden drop in blood pressure. The term "vagal" comes from the vagus nerve that passes through the body from the brain to the stomach and is responsible for slowing down cardiac activity when it accelerates. At idle, the heart brings less blood to the arteries, the brain is, therefore, less oxygenated, which results in a spontaneous loss of consciousness, but usually very brief.

Vagal discomfort is the most common form of fainting or fainting. Clinically, the biological process and mechanisms involved in this type of discomfort are well known, but not exhaustive.

Discomfort is one of the common problems currently facing cardiologists and general practitioners. Indeed, with an annual incidence (appearance of new cases of the pathology) of between 1.3 and 2.7 per 1,000 individuals, vagal discomfort should, therefore, be considered carefully.

Different forms of vagal discomfort exist:

- benign form, resulting in the form of syncope;
- the more serious form, affecting patients with underlying pathologies, such as heart abnormalities, neurological diseases, etc.
- Syncope, and therefore vagal discomfort, is defined as sudden and generally short-term loss of consciousness. The return to "normal state" is spontaneous and rapid. It is also characterized by global cerebral hypoperfusion. Or by the decrease in vascularity in the brain.

What should you do if you have vagal discomfort?

Nausea, dizziness, pale face, blurred vision, sweating, dry mouth, hot flushes, buzzing hearing, general weakening ... When a person is experiencing vagal discomfort, it is important to elevate his legs in order to oxygenate the brain to restore balance to the heart system.

If the person passes out, place them in the Lateral Safety Position (PLS). This first aid is used to clear the airways of the body.

If the person has not recovered quickly, the emergency services must be alerted immediately.

When you feel that you are having this kind of discomfort, try to lie down or squat down, if you are sitting, it is better to remain so and not to get up.

Some clues can help recognize vagal discomfort:

- ✓ hot flashes;
- ✓ nausea ;
- ✓ extreme fatigue;
- ✓ blurred vision;
- ✓ sweating;
- ✓ pallor;
- ✓ diarrhea;
- ✓ successive yawns;
- ✓ hearing impairment, such as tinnitus.

In most cases, vagal discomfort is not serious. However, the fall it causes is not without danger.

The causes are various, linked to hypersensitivity of the vagal nerve or to other external factors:

- ✓ period of intense stress
- ✓ overwork
- ✓ sensitivity, anxiety
- ✓ emotional shock

- ✓ hot weather
- ✓ feeling of compartmentalization
- ✓ phobias (blood, crowd, etc.)
- ✓ after local anesthesia
- ✓ taking certain medications, such as isoproterenol, nitroglycerin, or even clomipramine.

In other cases, the causes of vagal discomfort are not trivial. Neurobiological or cardiovascular disorders can occur.

In any case, a person prone to one or more vagal discomforts must consult a health professional. A diagnosis and an evaluation of the clinical case will make it possible to specify the cause of the discomfort. The healthcare professional will be particularly interested in the patient's history, lifestyle, and social context (family and professional situation, etc.).

What are the symptoms and treatment of vagal discomfort?

Little is known about the biological mechanisms involved in vagal discomfort. In addition, the brain has been shown to be strongly involved.

Vagal discomfort is then a "reflex" activation of the cerebral cortex, the triggering of which is rapid, inducing a decrease in the heart rate and a reduction in muscle tone.

Activation of these reflex mechanisms then causes

- ✓ bradycardia, slow heart rate;
- ✓ vasodilation, increased caliber of blood vessels;
- ✓ hypotension, abnormally low blood pressure.

Most people with vagal discomfort show significant signs: feelings of imbalance when standing, dizziness, headache, and "return to normal" after a few minutes.

In other cases, the discomfort may last longer. And in this context, loss of consciousness, caused by cerebral hypoperfusion, then leads to convulsive movements or even epileptic seizures.

Signs can call out before discomfort occurs, such as intense fatigue, muscle weakness, wet skin, visual disturbances, or even tinnitus.

Diagnosis and treatment of vagal discomfort

The diagnosis of vagal discomfort is made beforehand by questions about the patient and thorough medical examinations. Questions must also be asked in the context of this first phase of diagnosis, in particular, if the loss of consciousness is really linked to syncope, if the patient has underlying heart disease or if clinical information on the individual would eventually help guide the diagnosis.

Tools for the diagnosis of vagal discomfort allow their early identification, for example, recording systems to identify possible arrhythmias. After the first discomfort, an Electroencephalogram (ECG) is then performed.

As part of the management of vagal discomfort, short-term hospitalization is sometimes necessary.

The treatments associated with vagal risk consist of limiting recurrences of discomfort, and thus in reducing the risk of mortality. In fact, syncope can be additional risk factors for accidents at work, in the context of physical and/or sporting practice or simply in daily accidents.

How to prevent vagal discomfort?

Prevention with patient education is part of the initial treatment of the disease. Indeed, avoid "triggering" factors, such as places and times likely to trigger a situation of stress and risk of discomfort and but also learning the gestures to implement in stopping a syncopic episode.

Drug treatments are not necessarily prescribed in patients who have had only one or two syncopes. However, as part of a higher frequency of discomfort, treatments are available. Among these, beta-blockers, disopyramide, scopolamine, theophylline, and others.

Finally, the doctor is held responsible for the prevention of driving under the risk of fainting. Indeed, the syncopic risk can prove to be dangerous for car drivers, who can put the patient, himself, in danger but also others.

To prevent vagal discomfort, it is better to eat a healthy and balanced diet, sleep in sufficient quantity, and practice physical activity regularly.

People at risk

The elderly, as well as people with underlying pathologies, are more concerned with the risk of syncope. Indeed, high blood pressure, diabetes, or even aging interfere with the self-regulation of cerebral vascularization. In this sense, the risk of syncope is greater.

The incidence and prevalence are all the more important with age (from 70 years). In France, almost 1.2% of vagal discomfort cases result in urgent care. 58% of patients with this type of discomfort are hospitalized.

This syncope corresponds to a sudden and brief loss of consciousness. Often benign, it is due to excessive stimulation of the vegetative function of the vagus nerve, which is responsible for slowing the heart rate.

- Peptic ulcer. It results from an inflammation of the gastric wall (gastric ulcer) or duodenum, the first part of the intestine (duodenal ulcer). Gastric acid secretion, regulated by the vagus nerve, can promote the appearance of ulcers.
- Dysphonia. Speech disorders can be observed following a lesion of the vagus nerve, and more generally, of the pharyngeal branches.
- Epilepsy. It is characterized by abnormal nerve impulses in the brain.

Treatment of the vagus nerve

- Medical treatment. In the case of peptic ulcer, certain drugs can be prescribed to decrease the acidity and treat the infection: antibiotics, antihistaminics, antacids.

- Vagustomy. Performed if drug treatment is not enough in case of peptic ulcer, this surgical procedure consists of partially or totally cutting the vagus nerve in the abdomen.
- Speech therapy rehabilitation. In the case of dysphonia and if the nerve is not completely severed, speech therapy will be implemented.
- Surgical treatment. As a last resort, surgery will be performed.
- Stimulation of the vagus nerve. Depending on the diagnosis, different methods of stimulating the vagus nerve (vagal maneuvers) can be practiced.

Vagus nerve exams

- Physical examination. Studying the different symptoms can help identify vagus nerve damage.
- Electrophysiological exploration. The electromyogram is used to study the electrical activity of the vagus nerve and to identify potential lesions.
- Electrocardiogram: what is electrocardiogram?

The electrocardiogram is an examination that records the electrical activity of the heart as your heartbeats.

Indeed, the heart, like all muscles, contracts under the influence of successive electrical impulses (polarizations and repolarizations), which can be detected and recorded.

In reality, the electrocardiogram designates the plot of the electrical activity obtained; the test is called electrocardiography (ECG).

The ECG is an essential examination in cardiology. It can be prescribed in many situations:

- in case of chest pain
- to detect arrhythmias (heart rhythm disturbances)
- to detect other heart conditions such as coronary insufficiency (blockage of the arteries supplying the heart), the presence of

damaged areas in the heart (due to a lack of irrigation or a recent heart attack), dilation of the heart, etc.
- to monitor heart activity in case of known heart disease
- in case of emergency admission for chest pain
- during a preoperative assessment
- etc.

In all of these situations, the EKG is abnormal.

It is a non-invasive, painless exam.

The principle is simple. By sticking electrodes to the surface of the skin, on the thorax, it is possible to record the difference in "potential" (electrical difference) between two points diametrically opposite with respect to the heart, and therefore to record the electrical activity of the heart.

In practice, to perform an ECG, many electrodes are used (between 12 and 15), placed on the chest but also on the arms and legs.

If necessary, the skin is washed and dried beforehand, shaved, to allow better adhesion. The electrodes are fixed with adhesive patches.

The ECG is recorded, most often in the supine position, for 5-10 minutes, sometimes longer. The drawing is done automatically on a roll of paper, which is progressively unrolling.

What results can you expect from an EKG?

The normal ECG shows a so-called "sinus" trace, with different electrical periods.

The doctor will interpret the route obtained to detect any anomalies, which may relate to:

- frequency (normally between 60 and 100 beats per minute);
- the nature of the rhythm (for example absence of one of the normal elements of the curve);

- the amplitude of certain waves;
- the length of the interval between others.

Depending on the results, he can direct the diagnosis and request, if necessary, the completion of additional examinations such as an exercise ECG.

This test records the electrical activity of the heart to detect abnormalities.

- Medical imaging. Additional examinations can be performed to confirm the diagnosis: radiography, cerebral MRI, abdominal MRI, cerebral and spinal scanner, chest scanner, abdominal scanner etc.

History and symbolism of the vagus nerve

The discovery of acetylcholine, secreted during stimulation of the vagus nerve, has led to great progress in neurology, particularly in the understanding of neurotransmission. This medical revolution earned the two scientists Henry Hallet Dale and Otto Loewi the Nobel Prize in Physiology in 1936 "for their discoveries about the chemical transmission of nerve impulses."

CHIROPRACTICS FOR YOUR VAGUS NERVE

The importance of the vagus nerve

The vagus nerve is the tenth cranial nerve, and it has the most extensive distribution of all cranial nerves. Named for its tendency to "wander," it acts as a switchboard for neurological information, communicating most organs of the body with the brain. Its main function is to relax, activating the parasympathetic nervous system.

The vagus nerve leaves the skull through a small hole, and from there it reaches the ears, throat (pharynx and larynx), tongue, stomach, intestines, heart, liver, spleen, pancreas, gallbladder, kidneys and organs players.

The problems that result when the vagus nerve does not work properly are very numerous, and include anxiety and depression, ringing in the ears, difficulty swallowing, difficulty speaking, irritable bowel syndrome, gastroesophageal reflux, heartburn, and inflammatory bowel diseases, such as Crohn's disease and ulcerative colitis, among many others.

More recent research is documenting the importance of the vagus nerve for the functioning of the body. Vagal activation is associated with growth and weight gain in babies. Studies have shown that gastric motility stimulated by the vagus nerve produces better absorption of food and, consequently, greater weight gain. The vagus nerve controls heart rate and blood pressure. Vagal stimulation increases kidney filtration and sodium excretion, and as a consequence, blood pressure decreases. Activation of the vagus nerve releases acetylcholine, which helps decrease inflammation. In addition, the reproductive organs are influenced by the activation of the vagus nerve, which makes it a key part of fertility.

CHIROPRACTIC AND VAGUS NERVE.

How can chiropractic care promote vagal nerve?

Looking at the anatomy of the vagus nerve, we see that its path is made through the medullary bridge and the first vertebra (the atlas) where there are its ramifications towards the autonomous system. Thus we can quickly understand that a problem of vertebral subluxation at the occipitoatlantoaxial level of the spine can impair the normal motor function of the vagus nerve, causing a type of compression and its physiological consequences.

To adjust this segment of the atlas, several chiropractic techniques can be used, such as the wide-ranging biomechanical adjustment. Also, the Toggle Recoil developed by B.J Palmer of high speed and low force or, more energetic techniques such as Network Spinal Analysis of low amplitude and promoting mechanical and electromagnetic oscillations.

They all have the same goal that is to stimulate the vagal tone to reduce the inflammation process via the inhibition of cytokine production (the inflammatory reflex).

A recent study has demonstrated the effectiveness of chiropractic adjustments to increase the activity of the vagus nerve. Vagus nerve activation levels can be studied by measuring heart rate variability. Patients under regular chiropractic care showed better heart rate and adaptability than those who were not.

In another study, chiropractic adjustments have a very important influence on the nervous system. Using a positron emission tomography, they showed metabolic brain changes and an increase in activation of the vagus nerve after releasing vertebral nerve pressure with adjustments.

It is important to remember that the vagus nerve leaves the skull through a small hole between cranial bones. Tension in the skull, cervical, or upper back can alter the shape and position of this hole and cause nerve compression, decreasing its function.

The increase in vagal activity associated with chiropractic care is one of the mechanisms by which chiropractic promotes the health and well-being of families. This is the true power of chiropractic.

Here are some strategies to stimulate the activity of the vagus nerve:

- Cold. Wash your hands with cold water. Take a few minutes of a cold shower.
- Practice diaphragmatic breathing. Breathe slowly and deeply, feeling the belly rise. Make the expiration last as long as you can.
- Eat blue fish and seafood. They have essential omega-3 fatty acids necessary for the proper functioning of the vagus nerve.
- Massage the earlobe.
- Sing!
- Laughs loudly!

We know that inflammatory responses play a fundamental role in the development and persistence of many diseases and can lead to debilitating chronic pain.

In most cases, inflammation is the body's natural response to a type of stress. But if the chances of stress that cause the "fight or flight" reaction of the nervous system and, therefore, the less biological footprint of stressful stimuli, reduce inflammation, are reduced.

Anti-inflammatories are routinely prescribed to fight inflammation, but the evidence that vagus nerve stimulation and improvement of the "vagal tone" work is also increasing. A healthy and adequate "vagal tone" can be achieved through certain holistic therapies such as meditation, yoga, acupuncture, or chiropractic, among others.

What is the vagus nerve in other terms?

It is the cranial nerve X, from the Latin vagus or vagabond, which originates from the brainstem and has many branches of nerve fibers in the thoracic and abdominal cavity, with motor-sensory fibers in the heart, larynx, pharynx to the intestine.

In 1921, a German physiologist Otto Loewi discovered that stimulating the vagus nerve could reduce the heart rate, causing the secretion of a substance he called vagal substance ("vagusstoff" in German). Later, this substance was identified as acetylcholine and was the first neurotransmitter identified by scientists. This neurotransmitter is like a "tranquilizer" and can be secreted only by taking a deep breath! Simply activating the vagus nerve reflex consciously can produce a feeling of inner calm and decrease inflammation. The vagus nerve is an essential component of the parasympathetic nervous system that regulates the "rest and digestion" responses. In return, to maintain homeostasis, there is the sympathetic system that regulates the response of the "fight or flight."

A healthy vagal tone and positive emotions feed each other.

A deep diaphragmatic inhalation followed by a long exhalation is a key to stimulate the vagus nerve and slow heart rate and blood pressure.

The index of a high tone of the vagus nerve is related to physical and psychosocial well-being. And vice versa, a low index is related to inflammation and depression (2010 research, Barbara Frederikson and Bethany Kok of the University of North Carolina at Chapel Hill published in Psychological Science, "How positive emotions build psychic health")

In summary, the key to well-being would be to reduce this inflammatory reflex through the mechanical stimulation of the vagal tone and reducing the external factors of inflammation (physical, chemical, emotional, psychosocial, and electromagnetic).

CHIROPRACTICS ALSO HELPS DIGESTIVE DISORDER

More than 80 million dollars are spent each year on medications to relieve heartburn, acid reflux, bloating, gas, irritable bowel syndrome, constipation, diarrhea, and other digestive disorders. These symptoms that involve abnormal digestive functioning are becoming increasingly frequent in our society. Science and research have shown that chiropractic treatment offers a powerful solution to this modern epidemic.

The nervous system controls digestive function from different regions. The vagus nerve that starts from the brain stem and passes near the "Atlas" or first cervical innervates all the main organs of digestion and stimulates the digestive process. Other important areas that control the digestion process include the sympathetic nerves that leave the thoracic and lumbar regions and the parasympathetic sacral nerve fibers. Vertebral subluxations in any of these areas can lead to neurological compromise and alterations in digestive function.

Chiropractors look for the location of these subluxations. A specific chiropractic adjustment realigns the altered regions and restores the innervation of the affected organs. This approach enhances the body's innate ability and works to harmonize this incredible life force in order to improve organ function and quality of life.

Several studies have demonstrated the power of chiropractic adjustments in restoring optimal function in people with digestive disorders. In 2008 a study demonstrated the effectiveness of chiropractic adjustments in children with digestive problems. The researchers selected three children who had bowel movements with a frequency from once a week to once every 3 or 4 days. The parents of these children had tried different laxatives and other procedures recommended by doctors. He had also followed specific changes in diets and had taken cod liver oil and mineral oil without any results.

Children began receiving chiropractic adjustments for periods from 3 weeks to 3 months according to the study by author DR Larry S. Arbeitman, DC. "The three children experienced an almost immediate improvement. At the end of the study, the three had bowel movements at least once a day.

Subluxations in these specific areas of the spine can cause intestinal malfunction. Over the years, people of all ages have been seen who suffered from constipation for several days, feeling an improvement after an adjustment. Regular chiropractic adjustments can help patients establish a comfortable and effortless removal rate.

VAGUS NERVE STIMULATION

Vagus nerve electrostimulation involves using a device to stimulate the vagus nerve with electrical impulses. An implantable vagus nerve stimulator is currently approved by the Food and Drug Administration to treat epilepsy and depression. There is a vagus nerve on each side of the body, which extends from the brainstem, through the neck, to the chest and abdomen.

In conventional vagus nerve electrostimulation, a device is surgically implanted under the skin of the chest, and a wire is inserted under the skin, which connects the device to the left vagus nerve. When active, the device sends electrical signals along the nerve to the brainstem, which then sends signals to certain areas of the brain. The right vagus nerve is not used because it is more likely to contain fibers that supply the nerves of the heart.

New and non-invasive vagus nerve electrostimulation devices, which do not require surgical implantation, were approved in Europe to treat epilepsy, depression, and pain. The Food and Drug Administration (FDA) recently approved in the United States a non-invasive device that stimulates the vagus nerve for the treatment of headaches in salvas.

Approximately one-third of people with epilepsy do not respond fully to anticonvulsant medications. Vagus nerve stimulation may be an option to reduce the frequency of seizures in people who have not managed to control the condition with medication.

The Food and Drug Administration (FDA) approved vagus nerve stimulation for people who meet the following requirements:

- ✓ They are four years of age or older.
- ✓ They have focal epilepsy (partial).
- ✓ They have seizures that cannot be well controlled with medication.

In addition, the FDA approved vagus nerve stimulation for the treatment of depression in adults who meet the following requirements:

- They suffer from chronic depression and difficult to treat (treatment-resistant depression).
- They did not improve after trying four or more medications, with electroconvulsive therapy or both.
- They continue with standard treatments for depression, along with vagus nerve stimulation.

Risks

For most people, vagus nerve stimulation is safe. However, it presents some risks, both in surgery to implant the device and in brain stimulation.

Risks of the surgery

Surgical complications of the vagus nerve stimulation implant are rare and are similar to the dangers of other types of surgeries. For example:

- Pain in the area where the cut (incision) was made to implant the device

- Infection
- Difficulty to swallow
- Paralysis of the vocal cords, which is usually temporary, but can be permanent

Side effects after surgery

Some of the side effects and health problems associated with stimulation of the implanted vagus nerve may include the following:

- Voice changes
- Hoarseness
- Sore throat
- Cough
- Headaches
- Difficulty breathing
- Difficulty to swallow
- Itchy or tingling skin
- Insomnia
- Worsening sleep apnea

For most people, the side effects are tolerable. They may decrease over time, but some side effects may remain bothersome while using implanted vagus nerve stimulation.

Adjusting electrical impulses can help minimize these effects. If the side effects are intolerable, the device can be turned off temporarily or permanently.

How do you prepare

It is important to carefully consider the advantages and disadvantages of stimulating the implanted vagus nerve before deciding to undergo the procedure. Make sure you know all the other treatment options and that both you and the doctor consider that implanted vagus nerve stimulation is the best option for you. Ask the doctor what exactly to expect during surgery and after the pulse generator is in place.

Food and medicine

You may need to stop certain medications in advance, and your doctor may ask you not to eat the night before the procedure.

What you can expect

Before the procedure

You may need to have blood tests or other tests to make sure you don't have any health problems that could cause a problem. Your doctor may ask you to start taking antibiotics before surgery to prevent infections.

During the procedure

Surgery to implant the vagus nerve stimulation device can be performed on an outpatient basis, although some surgeons recommend spending the night in the hospital.

Generally, the surgery lasts from one hour to an hour and a half. You can stay awake and receive medication to anesthetize the surgery area (local anesthesia), or you may be unconscious during the surgery (general anesthesia).

The surgery itself does not compromise the brain. Two incisions are made, one in the chest or in the region of the armpit (axillary) and the other in the left side of the neck.

The pulse generator is implanted in the upper left side of the chest. The device is intended as a permanent implant but can be removed if necessary.

The pulse generator is about the size of a stopwatch and is battery operated. In the pulse generator, a conductor cable is connected. This cable is guided under the skin, from the chest to the neck, where it joins the vagus nerve through a second incision.

After the procedure

The pulse generator is turned on during a visit to the doctor's office a few weeks after surgery. Then it can be programmed to send electrical impulses to the vagus nerve with different durations, frequencies, and currents. Usually, vagus nerve stimulation begins at a low level and gradually increases, depending on your symptoms and side effects.

Stimulation is programmed to turn on and off in specific cycles, for example, 30 seconds on and 5 minutes off. You may have some tingling sensations or slight neck pain and temporary hoarseness when nerve stimulation is activated.

When activated, the stimulator turns on and off according to the intervals the doctor selected. You can use a hand-magnet to start stimulation at a different time, for example, if you perceive an impending attack.

You should visit the doctor periodically to make sure that the pulse generator is working properly and that it has not run out of position. Consult with your doctor before undergoing any medical test, such as magnetic resonance imaging (MRI), which could interfere with your device.

Results

Implantation of the implanted vagus nerve is not a cure for epilepsy. Most people with epilepsy will not stop having seizures or taking medication against epilepsy after the procedure. However, many of them will have fewer seizures, up to 20 to 50 percent less. The intensity of seizures may also decrease.

It may take months or even a year or more of the stimulation before you notice any considerable reduction in seizures. Vagus nerve stimulation can also shorten the recovery time after a seizure. People who have undergone vagus nerve stimulation to treat epilepsy may also experience improvements in mood and quality of life.

Research is not yet definitive in terms of the benefits of implanted vagus nerve stimulation to treat depression. As suggested in some studies, the benefits of vagus nerve stimulation for depression accumulate over time, and it may take several months of treatment before you notice any improvement in depression symptoms. Implantation of the implanted vagus nerve does not work in all cases and is not intended to replace traditional treatments.

Also, some health insurance companies may not cover this procedure.

The autonomic nervous system takes care of all the automatic tasks in our bodies. There is the sympathetic nervous system, which is the accelerator and the parasympathetic, the brake. The parasympathetic takes care of rest and digestion, repair while the sympathetic system is for activity, it is the master of the fight or flees response.

The enteric nervous system is sometimes integrated into the autonomic nervous system or as a separate entity, but in reality, they are intimately linked.

The vagus nerve monitors almost the entire body, sending information about the state of the organs. It innervates the brain, spine, tongue, pharynx, vocal cords, lungs, heart, stomach, intestines and glands that produce enzymes and anti-stress hormones (such as acetylcholine, prolactin, vasopressin, oxytocin), it controls mood, heart rate, digestion, respiration, immune response, etc.

Too much stress, be it physical, biological, toxic, chemical, emotional, or psychological, acts strongly on the activity of the vagus nerve, the tenth cranial nerve.

When the sympathetic system flares up, the tone of the vagus nerve decreases.

80% of messages go from the gut to the brain and the digestive system - directly linked to different areas of the brain by the vagus nerve - sends the messages in milliseconds.

Food, microbial, and inflammatory factors modulate the gut-brain axis and influence physiological processes ranging from metabolism to cognition.

THE POTENTIAL OF THE VAGUS NERVE

More and more research is being done on the stimulation of the vagus nerve, which increases its tone, has anti-inflammatory properties, and allows neuroimmune communication in the intestine.

It decreases allergic-type reactions.

The brain-gut axis is becoming increasingly important as a therapeutic target for gastrointestinal and psychiatric disorders, such as inflammatory bowel disease, depression, and post-traumatic stress disorder.

Stimulation of the vagus nerve in the gut influences the monoaminergic brain systems of the brainstem, which play a crucial role in major psychiatric disorders, such as mood and anxiety disorders. (R) (R) A system which I already mentioned in a previous article Warrior gene, monoamine oxidase: towards an increasingly violent world or even in this article The blocking of an enzyme involved in addictions

According to Stephen Porges, author of "The polyvagal theory": "The swinging and swinging behaviors commonly seen in people with autism may reflect a natural bio-behavioral strategy to stimulate and regulate a vagal system that is not working effectively. Living things from the inside, I know that I had often used different behavioral behaviors against anxiety, like humming, which was interpreted as a sign of joy when it was the opposite.

A damaged vagus nerve cannot send signals to your abdominal muscles. This can cause food to stay longer in your stomach, rather than moving normally through your small intestine for digestion, which is part of the GERD reflux complex.

The vagus nerve is the central control for the functioning of our parasympathetic nervous system and uses acetylcholine to communicate.

It is interesting to note that mercury blocks the action of acetylcholine and that it is one of the heaviest pollutions with 3000 tons of mercury spread in the atmosphere every year. Aluminum is recognized as neurotoxic and, more particularly, for the cholinergic system. (R) (R) No wonder it is linked to various pathologies such as Alzheimer's, autism, fibromyalgia, etc.

The vagus nerve may no longer react to stimuli; it is then hypotonic or, on the contrary, react excessively and be hypertonic.

When the vagus nerve is under-reactive, it often causes a condition called gastroparesis, which is a common and serious complication of diabetes. Patients with this disorder may experience stomach pain, nausea, heartburn, spasms, and weight loss. Patients with underactive vagal nerves often experience serious gastrointestinal problems. People whose vagus nerve is too active may pass out.

Any type of gastrointestinal distress can put pressure on and irritate the nerve, often caused by hiatal hernia.

Any stress, whether physical, chemical or psychological can ignite the Yoga and moderate exercise

Yoga is associated with elevated mood and reduced anxiety, increasing GABA levels, and the activity of the parasympathetic system. In response to light physical exercise, the vagal nerve stimulates gastric motility and improves the stomach's ability to process food. This is why we talk about digestive walking.

Massages

- Massages of the neck or feet can increase the tone of the vagus nerve.
- Calorie restriction or intermittent fasting
- The calorie restriction that shows multiple benefits activates the parasympathetic system.
- Sleep on the right side
- To activate your vagus nerve, choose to lie on your right side.

We cannot imagine how important all this is, and according to the way I look at the world, regaining knowledge of ourselves so that we can make an inner revolution is the most important. A particular vision that I reveal in my second work, "Living Through Heaven or Science? " Because a healthy vagus nerve achieves the balance between the sympathetic and parasympathetic nervous system and what is called The ANS is a very small brain on its own, its name "autonomous" comes from the fact that it ensures bodily functions without our consciousness or control (without conscious participation on our part).

The ANS is divided into two parts, the sympathetic system, and the parasympathetic system. These two systems often act in an opposite way (antagonist) what makes that the physical state represents at every moment the balance between the two systems: it is homeostasis.

Homeostasis is a system of self-regulation of our vital bodily functions. It is thanks to this system that we humans have survived to this day.

Good homeostasis allows the almost immediate adaptation of the heart rate according to needs, the provision of the right amount of blood and oxygen. Imagine that you have to run fast all of a sudden, if your system does not provide the necessary blood and oxygen, you will pass out and vice versa if the system produces an influx of blood and oxygen too abundant compared to the needs of the moment, you will also feel bad.

So homeostasis is a very subtle balance, which must be able to adapt quickly to the demands of the situation.

Controlled by the hypothalamus, the SNA organizes homeostasis in a coordinated manner. Homeostasis means maintaining the "status quo" in the human system. Thus, blood pressure, body temperature, fluid and electrolyte balance, as well as body weight, are kept at a precise value, the reference value (normal).

To be able to perform its tasks, the hypothalamus must constantly receive information on the state of the body and be able to trigger compensatory changes if a value deviates from its "normal" value.

To solve a problem that arises, the hypothalamus has two solutions to choose from:

1. Sending signals to the ANS (by the nerves, i.e. neurological which means electrical) By sending these signals through the spinal cord, it controls vital functions such as heart rate, vasoconstriction (i.e., tone), digestion, sweating, etc.

2. Sending endocrine signals (by hormones, i.e. chemical)

These signals are sent to the pituitary gland, which routes them to the various endocrine glands in the body.flow or the state of grace and spontaneous joy.

The role of the vagus nerve in the relaxation response

The vagus nerve has many functions, but some of the most important is due to its role as a major component of the autonomic nervous system. This system controls involuntary bodily functions, such as heart rate, digestion, and breathing.

The autonomic nervous system is divided into two main branches, the parasympathetic and the sympathetic nervous system. The sympathetic nervous system prepares the body to deal with the perceived danger when initiating the fight or flight stress response.

On the contrary, the parasympathetic nervous system prepares the body for rest. This relaxed state should be your default state, but in people with problems with stress or anxiety, it may not be the case. The vagus nerve is the main conduit of the parasympathetic nervous system. In addition to initiating the relaxation response, the nerve also influences the reduction of inflammation, memory storage, and the maintenance of the body in a state of balance called homeostasis. In addition, the vagus nerve causes the production of many important neurotransmitters, especially GABA, norepinephrine, and acetylcholine.

Signs and symptoms of vagus nerve dysfunction

The health and function of the vagus nerve are closely related to the vagal tone. When the vagus nerve is functioning as it should, it is said that it has a high vagal tone. High vagal tone is related to good physical health, mental well-being, and stress resistance.

When the vagus nerve is not working as well as it should, it has a low vagal tone. People who get stressed easily and have trouble calming down after experiencing stress may have a low vagal tone.

Since one of the many functions of the vagus nerve is to act as a switch for inflammation, the low vagal tone often leads to chronic inflammation, an important factor in many diseases of the body and mind, including ADHD, anxiety, depression, Alzheimer's, heart disease, cancer, and diabetes. In addition, the low vagal tone has been linked to a long list of physical and mental health conditions that range from mild to severe.

The influence of vagal tone on health is widespread and affects many important systems. Hence, some symptoms and disorders related to low vagal tone are the following:

- Constipation.
- Depression.
- Diabetes.
- Anxiety disorders
- Autoimmune disorders
- Bipolar disorder.
- Difficulty to swallow.
- Tendency to choke on eating.
- Digestive disorders, included gastroparesis.
- Hoarseness.
- Migraines
- Obesity.
- Rheumatoid arthritis.
- Sudden increases in blood pressure.

- Heart disease (increased heart rate).
- Addictions
- Alzheimer disease.
- Chronic Fatigue Syndrome.
- Epilepsy.

KEYS TO STIMULATE THE VAGUS NERVE

There are many ways to stimulate the vagus nerve to keep the vague tone high and healthy. Researchers use the term vagus nerve modulation more accurately, which means the ability to regulate or balance. Thus, what stimulates the vagus nerve is actually what tones and strengthens it, just as exercise tones and strengthens your muscles.

A healthier vagus nerve is more receptive, which helps you recover from stress more quickly.

STIMULATE THE VAGUS NERVE USING THE MIND-BODY CONNECTION

- Some exercises and body-mind therapies that help improve the tone of the vagus nerve are the following:
- Sing. Singing alone or with others stimulates the vagus nerve, according to research. When singing with other people, the heart rate is synchronized. It is believed that the vagus nerve is responsible for this.
- To meditate. One study found that meditating autonomously helped tone the vagus nerve. In addition, it has been discovered that OM singing increases vagal tone while reducing activity in the amygdala, the fear center of the brain.
- Yoga. Moderate exercise of any kind can stimulate the vagus nerve, but yoga stands out above all of them. Numerous studies support that yoga increases the parasympathetic activity of the nervous system, which, in turn, improves vagal tone. For example, one study found that yoga not only improves vagal tone but also increased the release of GABA, the neurotransmitter of relaxation.

- Acupuncture. Strengthens the vagal tone. Traditional acupuncture points, particularly atrial acupuncture, stimulate the vagus nerve, as research has shown.
- Reflexology. It has been found that foot reflexology increases vagal tone.

VAGUS NERVE AND SLEEP.

The stimulation of the vagus nerve is a validated technique in the management of drug-resistant epilepsies.

Its mode of action remains undetermined in epilepsy but seems to involve key structures known for their role in sleep (solitary tract, crosslinked substance).

The effect of stimulation of the vagus nerve differs depending on the intensity, frequency of stimulation, and the time elapsed since it was started and is generally beneficial for the quality of sleep.

It can, however, aggravate or facilitate the appearance of a sleep apnea syndrome, the latter must, therefore, be systematically sought beforehand in any candidate for stimulation of the vagus nerve.

OTHER WAYS TO STIMULATE THE VAGUS NERVE

healthy relationship is a key to maintaining the health of the vagus nerve. In fact, it is known that people with a better vagal tone are more altruistic and have closer and more harmonious relationships.

This is partly because vagal stimulation causes the release of oxytocin, a hormone called "connection molecule," because it promotes binding. Oxytocin has been linked to human traits such as loyalty, empathy, trust, and courage.

In this sense, research has discovered that there is a cycle of positive feedback between edifying social connections, positive emotions, and physical health set in motion by the vagal tone.

Therefore, one way to stimulate the vagus nerve is to meet friends to laugh with. Laughter strengthens relationships while increasing heart rate variability, a reliable indicator of the healthy function of the vagus nerve.

Finally, another way to stimulate the vagus nerve is worth mentioning: through supplements. Some supplements can improve the health and function of the vagus nerve, such as ginger root, probiotics (specifically Lactobacillus rhamnosus), essential omega-3 fatty acids (especially DHA), and zinc.

CHAPTER THREE

HOW TO STIMULATE THE VAGUS NERVE TO RELIEVE STRESS AND IMPROVE THE FUNCTIONING OF THE BODY

Learn how you can help your body relieve tensions and relax by stimulating the vagus nerve.

Our body forms a whole in an integral way. Each termination joins with another in a network of connections that would explain why a point pain could be caused by a condition in another region that seems to be totally disconnected.

Just as in our body, we have nerves that are born from the spinal cord, inside the spine, and transmit the sensory and motor impulses to the brain; We also have twelve pairs of nerves that emerge from the skull and specifically control the region of the neck and face.

One of them, the one that occupies the tenth pair, is what is known as the vagus nerve, one of the longest in the body since it extends from the skull to the abdomen.

This nerve is the main parasympathetic nervous system, which is responsible for facilitating the functions that allow the body to relax, unlike the "sympathetic" that is the one that motorizes the necessary mechanisms to maintain the alert state.

In this way, the vagus nerve allows, after having been more active, the heart rate becomes slower, blood pressure decreases, the body relaxes, and digestion and sleep are regulated. The neurotransmitter that causes these nerves to activate is acetylcholine, a natural relaxant that can be activated through breathing, as you can see later.

Learning how to stimulate this nerve not only favors relaxation but also strengthens immune functions, helps reduce anxiety (and so it can also favor those who are overweight), to treat tachycardia, hypertension, and depression, among others sufferings

If we want to go deep, the vagus nerve provides nerve fibers to the throat, lungs, heart, digestive, and respiratory system. In addition, it controls muscle movement.

Therefore, if it is affected, there may be some symptoms such as gastrointestinal disorders (gas, inflammation, constipation, diarrhea, abdominal pain), anxiety, anger, depression without reason or disproportionate, reluctance, difficulty moving the tongue, arrhythmia, between others.

A very simple technique that you can perform anywhere is to make a conscious breath. This is the only function of the autonomic nervous system that can be regulated and promotes relaxation, elimination of toxins, concentration, and calm.

To perform abdominal or diaphragmatic breathing, you should only:

- Inspire through the nose slowly, mentally counting to 4.
- Hold the air in the lungs, counting to 6 and contracting the abdomen.
- Exhale counting to 4, slightly contracting the lips.

Try to do this several times every day and, especially in a stressful situation. Do it slowly and deeply, becoming aware of air travel throughout the body.

In addition to contributing to relaxation, this exercise, in the long term, can help lower blood pressure, improve heart rate, improve immune function, and reduce anxiety.

- Place a damp and fresh cloth on the face.
- Drink a glass of cold water quickly.
- Lie on an inclined surface, head down.

Take a diet that contains vegetables, nuts, and fruits, avoiding excess cereals (especially refined ones), oxidized vegetable oils, sugars, dairy products, and processed food. Keep in mind that your body has a great capacity for healing. Learn to work with him, and increase your ability to register to understand what may be happening to you and know when to turn in search of a professional who can help you.

HOW TO STIMULATE THE VAGUS NERVE TO INCREASE MENTAL AND BODY HEALTH

The vagus nerve is the longest and most complex nerve in the body. It connects the brain to many important organs throughout the body, including the intestine (intestines, stomach), heart, and lungs.

The vagus nerve is also a key part of the parasympathetic nervous system and influences breathing, digestive function, and heart rate, in addition to having an influence on mental health. Therefore, the optimization of the function of the vagus nerve can improve our health, strengthening our defenses against stress.

Increased vagal tone activates the parasympathetic nervous system. Having a superior vagal tone means that your body can relax faster after stress.

In fact, in 2010, researchers discovered a positive feedback loop between high vagal tone, positive emotions, and good physical health.

CHAPTER FOUR
RELEVANCE OF VAGUS NERVE STIMULATION

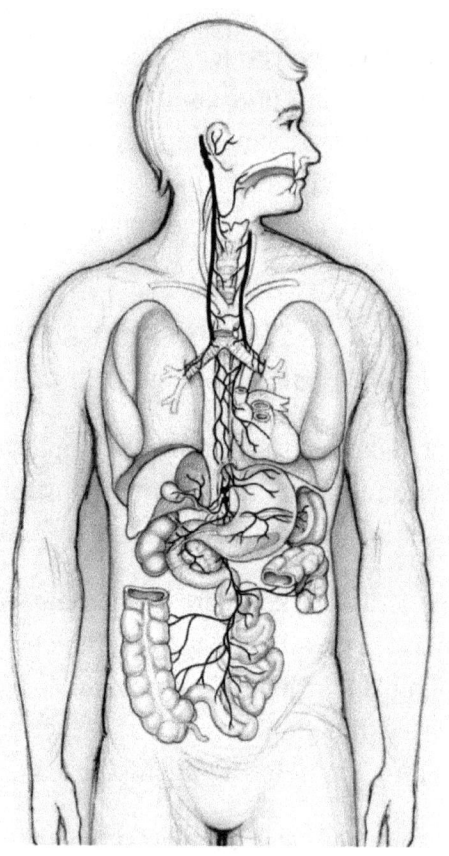

What does the vagus nerve do?

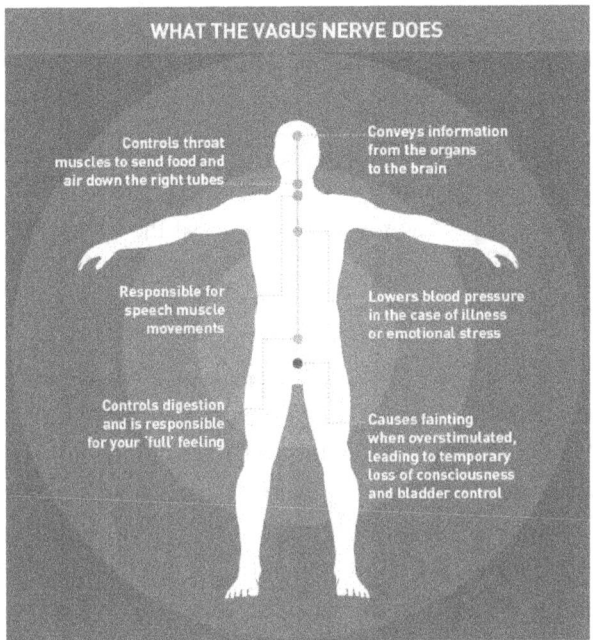

The vagus nerve (NV) originates from the brainstem, the trunk of the brain that detects, processes, and regulates the vast majority of automatic functions of the body. In general terms, we do not have to think about these functions to carry them out consciously. These functions are autonomous and are regulated by our system.

The term vagus derives from a Latin word that means "wandering, wandering, going from one place to another" and, to a lesser extent, "uncertain or vague." Given the extensive and imprecise nature of the nerve after an initial examination, anatomists and researchers searched for a descriptive word that would mean exactly this. When they decided on the term "vague," they called the nerve "vagabond."

Some of the functions that regulate the autonomic nervous system are the following:

- Heartbeats
- Blink
- Rate and respiratory depth

- Contraction and dilation of blood vessels
- Detoxification of the liver and kidneys
- Digestion in the digestive tract
- Open and close the sweat glands
- Produce saliva and tears
- Dilation and contraction of the pupils of the eyes
- Sexual excitement
- To pee

Within the brainstem, there are several groups of neuronal cell bodies called nuclei. Here, neurons assimilate information from other cells spread throughout the body. These nuclei have different functions and have names derived from Latin. The cores resemble a router in a home Internet connection. Some of the information enters the router through the connection of your cables or telephone line, the information is processed in the router, and it sends other information to your computer, your TV and other electronic devices connected to your network.

There are two main types of neurons that send information in one of two directions. The first is afferent neurons, which receive information about what happens inside and around your body. Afferent neurons receive information from the body to the brain, called afferent information. The second are called efferent neurons, which send information with regulatory or motor effects (called efferent information) to various organs and structures in the body so that efferent information is transmitted from the brain to the body.

The vagus nerve is connected to four nuclei within the brainstem. 80% of the information transmitted through the NV is afferent information, which means that the direction in which the information usually flows in the NV is from the organs of the body to the brain. The remaining 20% of the neurons in the NV transmit efferent information, from the brain to the body, causing certain functions to be carried out in each cell and each organ. It is interesting to verify that most medical students are shocked that only 20% of the function.

NV is efferent since it has so many efferent effects on the organs: imagine the amount of information that this nerve transmits to the brain, more than four times all the information transmitted from it.

Like the computer cables that you have at home, the groups of neurons within your nerves send information through them through electrical signals, which, upon reaching the end of the nerve, causing a chemical signal called a neurotransmitter to be released... These neurotransmitters bind to receptors in the cells that receive the signals, which produces an effect on the cells located at the end of the connection. The main neurotransmitter used by NV is acetylcholine (ACh), which has a powerful anti-inflammatory effect on the body.

Controlling the inflammatory system is one of the most important functions of NV; It is the main system of inflammatory control of the body and has powerful effects on your personal health and diseases. Many of the health disorders my patients suffer are due to high levels of inflammation in certain organs and systems, from the digestive tract to the liver and even the brain.

Inflammation is an important response within the body to keep us safe from bacterial and viral invaders, physical trauma, and other things that should not be present in the body. When the levels of inflammation are not controlled and become chronic, the effects can be serious and cause numerous health problems. Among the most common disorders related to high levels of inflammation are:

- Alzheimer disease
- Arthritis
- Asthma
- Cancer
- Crohn's disease
- Diabetes
- Coronary heart disease
- Hypertension
- High cholesterol
- Postural orthostatic tachycardia syndrome (POTS)

- Ulcerative colitis
- And any disorder that ends in the suffix "itis."

Most organs affected in these diseases are innervated (or connected) by the NV. Therefore, it is not only possible but more than likely that the NV does not work at an optimal level and does not have an anti-inflammatory effect on these organs, causing chronic inflammation and certain diseases.

It is important to remember that these disorders do not occur in isolation, and if one of them is present, it is likely that there is another. The same signals are sent through the vagus nerve to and from virtually every internal organ, so that if the levels of inflammation in an organ are not controlled, the same may happen in other areas.

Do you know the importance of the vagus nerve for your health?

It is responsible for connecting the brain with the main vital organs and control all involuntary acts of the organism

Have you ever wondered why your body performs various vital activities unconsciously without you being able to control them? The response is the vagus nerve. It receives this curious name because it is the one that controls the involuntary functions and acts of the body, such as breathing, blood circulation, or heartbeat. You may have heard about it on some occasions, but you may not be very clear about its important function within the body. It is part of the so-called cranial nerves and is one of the main motors of the autonomic nervous system at the parasympathetic (involuntary) level.

It is one of the longest nerves and connects the brain with various vital organs - among which the heart, bronchi, stomach, esophagus, intestine, pancreas and liver - and is responsible for the sensitivity of the tonsils, the back of the nose and the pharynx, the ear, and the larynx. Without a doubt, a fundamental element in the correct functioning of the organism. Do you want to know more about him?

Controls the functioning of vital organs

- Cardiovascular. Its effects on the heart include the decrease in heart rate and blood pressure.
- Respiratory. It facilitates the contraction of the bronchi and increases its secretions.
- Gastrointestinal. Increases gastric motility (ability to move spontaneously and independently) and intestinal activity, in addition to relaxing the sphincters.
- Urinary. Participates in the control of urination, favoring the expulsion of urine.
- Hormonal It also influences other metabolic functions, controlling, for example, thyroid or insulin secretion by the pancreas.

Favors calm

Its functioning can also affect mental health, especially as it affects stress and anxiety. The expert points out that there are studies that suggest that greater activity of the vagus nerve (due to its parasympathetic function) is associated with a situation of calm and energy reserve. This is mainly due to a lower heart rate, lower blood pressure, a calmer breathing pattern, and a lower excitation brain activity.

How to keep it fit?

Seeing all these factors, it is very clear the importance of proper functioning of the vagus nerve. This can be affected by various diseases such as some types of tumors and trauma that can cause compression during its journey; brain ailments located in the brain stem (such as stroke); some autoimmune and neurodegenerative pathologies; or diabetes mellitus. Dr. Portilla indicates that his injury can cause pain in the throat, difficulty swallowing, disorders in the circulatory regulation (with poor control of blood pressure and heart rate), loss of consciousness, nausea, vomiting, weight loss, constipation and retention of urine.

However, there are techniques to facilitate stimulation. From the medical point of view, there are various electrical devices that can be applied externally or by surgery and that are used in diseases such as epilepsy, migraine, and depression, among others. Although the doctor insists that there are no studies to ensure its effectiveness, some of the recommendations for his care include avoiding exposure to irritating external factors (such as the abuse of cold drinks), exercising it through deep and slow breathing, as well as diaphragmatic and some types of massages.

WHERE IS THE VAGUS NERVE LOCATED?

The longest nerve in the body is the vagus nerve. Without going into too many technical details, I want to explain where the nerve begins and how it runs and reaches the organs it innervates and how it sends information from one side to another. Let's follow its course through the body.

Brain stem connections

The neurons that form the vagus nerve begin in the brainstem, from four distinct nuclei. These nuclei consist of the dorsal motor nucleus, the solitary nucleus, the spinal trigeminal nucleus, and the ambiguous nucleus. Each of these nuclei controls the specific nerve component fibers.

Sensory neurons transmit signals from the skin that the vagus nerve innervates the trigeminal spinal nucleus. This includes a specific section of ear skin, which is important when activating the vagus nerve using an acupuncture treatment that we will discuss in later chapters. The signals from the internal organs of the body are transmitted to the solitary nucleus through the vagus nerve and transferred to the brain to process them. These signals include those of the stomach, intestinal tract, lungs, heart, liver, gallbladder, pancreas, and spleen. We can also send direct signals to these organs through the vagus nerve using parasympathetic fibers that originate in the dorsal motor nucleus. These signals help calm and regulate the function of the heart and lungs and increase the action of the intestine and intestinal tract, liver, pancreas, gallbladder, and spleen.

The last core that provides fibers to the NV is the ambiguous core. This nucleus has neurons that fulfill a motor function, which works specifically to control the majority of muscles present in the throat and upper respiratory tract. These muscles are responsible for keeping the airways open and producing sounds through the vocal cords, creating your voice.

The right and left vagus nerve are the only nerves in the body that have four different functions and four nuclei that specifically provide the fiber component. Most of the other nerves in the body transmit simple sensory information of the skin and motor signals for muscle movement. This distinction should make you understand how important the vagus nerve is and the magnitude of its function.

Now, let's follow the course of the nerves from the brainstem down to the neck, the chest (chest area), and the abdomen (abdomen area).

Inside the neck

From the area of the brainstem known as the oblong medulla or spinal bulb, the fibers to the left and right of the vagus nerve extend into the cranial cavity (inside the skull) and converge to form what we call the vagus nerve. The nerve then leaves the skull through an opening called the jugular foramen. This opening consists of a wide space that allows the nerve and other blood vessels to pass between the neck and the skull. Once the NV leaves the skull, it penetrates the upper area of the neck just behind the ear, between the internal jugular vein and the internal carotid artery. These blood vessels constitute direct blood lines to and from the brain and are extremely important in keeping us alive.

Being so close to these specific blood vessels indicates how important the vagus nerve is since any physical damage to these three structures can cause irreparable damage. In the case of blood vessels, damage can lead directly to death, while nerve damage leads to a total lack of function in many organs of the body.

Immediately after the vagus nerve passes through the jugular foramen, we observe a thickening of the nerve called the upper ganglion (or jugular ganglion). A ganglion is a thickening of a nerve formed by a series of cellular bodies of sensory neurons located very close to each other. The cellular bodies of the sensory nerves congregate in this ganglion and subsequently re-form in the thinnest section of the nerve, where the first branch of the vagus nerve originates.

The first branch of the NV is the atrial branch. The atrial branch passes back and penetrates the skull through an opening called the mastoid canaliculus, and enters the ear through another opening in the skull called the tympanomastoid fissure. The nerve extends to the skin of each ear. This branch feels touch, temperature, and moisture in the skin of the ear; specifically, the external canal, the swallow, and the atrium. It is the main target in the treatment of activation of NV dysfunction using atrial acupuncture (acupuncture points in the ear), which we will discuss in later chapters.

When the nerve begins to run down (or inferiorly, to use anatomical language), from the upper ganglion, the NV thickens again to form the lower ganglion, also known as the nodes node. This ganglion houses the cell bodies of neurons involved in transmitting information from internal organs. The nerve then returns to thin and immediately penetrates a duct created by a thickening of connective tissue called the carotid sheath. Together with the internal carotid artery and the internal jugular vein, the nerve

It has additional soft tissue protection as it descends through the neck.

Within the carotid sheath, the vagus nerve extends its next branch: the pharyngeal branch. The pharyngeal branch has neurons of the vagus nerve, but it also carries contributing neurons of the ninth and eleventh cranial nerves (glossopharyngeal nerve and accessory nerve). When these neurons converge, they pass towards the midline of the body until they reach the upper part of the throat, called the pharynx. In the pharynx, the vagus nerve emits motor signals to multiple muscles involved in the swallowing reflex, controlling the opening and closing of the upper respiratory tract and maintaining the gag or pharyngeal reflex.

As the vagus nerve descends down the sides of the neck inside the carotid sheath, it extends its third branch, known as the superior laryngeal nerve. This nerve branches off the NV shortly after the pharyngeal branch and sends motor signals to the muscles of the larynx on the vocal cords, specifically the muscles that control the tone of your voice.

As the NV runs down through the carotid sheath, it extends the cervical cardiac branches, which are two of the three branches that innervate the heart. The third branch, the thoracic, cardiac branch, originates shortly after leaving the carotid sheath in the chest area (chest). These branches intermingle with the nerves of the sympathetic nervous system and form the cardiac plexus (a plexus is a collection of nerve fibers from different branches and nerves of different origins that run to a specific location). We have two cardiac plexuses: one in front of the aorta, called the superficial cardiac plexus, and one behind the aortic arch, called the deep cardiac plexus. (The aorta is the main blood vessel, which carries blood from the heart to the rest of the body.)

in relation to the heart. For now, the most important thing to keep in mind is that these fibers control the frequency of electrical activity that pumps your heart.

Inside the thorax

After the nerve leaves the lower part of the sheath, it runs down and penetrates the thorax, behind the first and second ribs, and in front of the large blood vessels that extend from the heart.

The left vagus nerve passes in front of (before) the aortic arch and then extends its fourth branch: the recurrent laryngeal nerve. On the opposite side of the body, the right vagus nerve follows a similar path; however, it passes in front of the right subclavian artery and then extends its fourth branch, the right side of the recurrent laryngeal nerve.

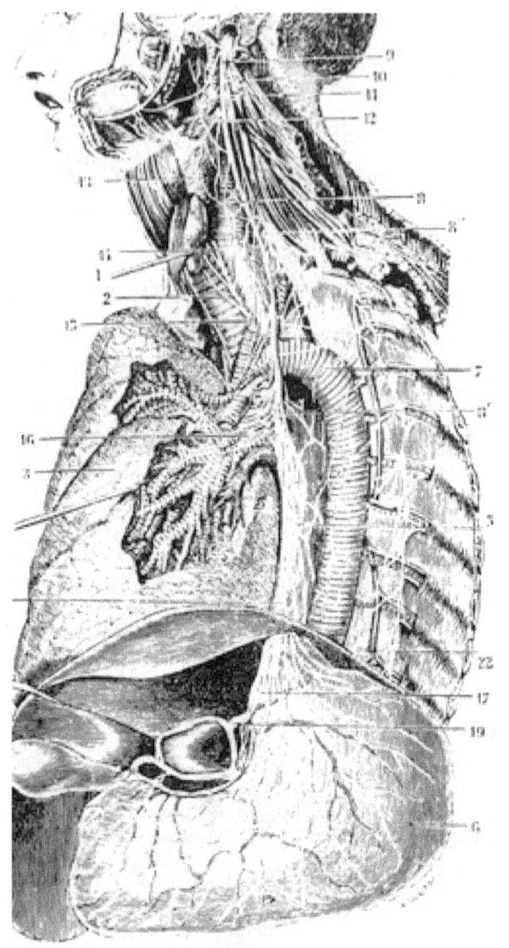

Both recurrent laryngeal nerves follow a similar path, but on opposite sides of the body. These are the only branches of the nerve that rotate and run upward again towards the neck. They carry motor signals from the brainstem to each of the laryngeal muscles below the vocal cords, which are important for the production of vocal sounds, based on the tension and relaxation of the vocal cords. Later we will abound in how we can use these specific branches to help improve the vagus nerve if it does not work optimally.

When the nerves reach the level of the aorta, each of the vagus nerves extends some branches to the next pair of organs: the lungs. The left vagus nerve sends a pulmonary branch to the anterior pulmonary plexus, and the right vagus nerve sends a pulmonary branch to the posterior pulmonary plexus. These nerve branches mix with the neurons of the sympathetic nervous system, reorganize and move to each side to innervate the lungs

Some fibers of the cardiac plexus extend to the sinoatrial nodule (SA) of the heart, while others extend to the atrioventricular nodule (AV).

These branches extend to the bronchi and major branches of the lungs to open and close them according to the body's need depending on each situation.

The thorax contains an organ innervated by the vagus nerve that is often overlooked and even forgotten: the thymus. The thymus is an extremely important organ of the immune system. It is located in the mediastinum of the chest, in front of the heart, but behind the sternum. A branch of the bum runs to this nerve and sends signals to and from the thymus. The thymus forms early in our development and is the main source of instruction and growth of our white blood cells. The reason we forget this organ so easily is that it shrinks over time and is replaced by fatty tissue. This process begins at puberty and can last many years until the beginning of adulthood. I consider the thymus a school for new immune cells, and as the school ages and deteriorates, the instruction that white blood cells get decreases in quality. In later chapters, we will abound in the role of the scam.

Inside the abdomen

The final section that innervates the vagus nerve is the organs of the abdomen. These organs are important for digestion, control the immune system, and ensure that the blood that reaches the rest of our cells does not contain toxins that can negatively affect cellular health.

The first abdominal branch of the vagus nerve extends to the stomach. When our body is in a state of rest-and-digestion, the vagus nerve fibers stimulate the stomach muscles to function. They send signals to the parietal cells to produce and secrete hydrochloric acid (HCl), the main cells that produce and secrete the digestive enzymes pepsin and gastrin, and to the smooth muscle cells of the stomach to agitate and physically boost the food in our stomach towards the next section of the digestive tract: the small intestine.

If the vagus nerve is damaged and does not send these important signals to the stomach cells, it causes problems such as hypochlorhydria, or low production of gastric acid, which is one of the main causes of numerous disorders. A sufficiently low pH (high acidity) is required to activate digestive enzymes and break down food. The optimal range of stomach pH should be around 3.0 in the stomach, while nothing above 5.0 will be powerful enough to activate pepsin and gastrin. The low production of gastric acid causes food degradation to be poor. A high pH in the stomach can also create bacteria, viruses, and unwanted parasites that penetrate the intestines and wreak havoc on the digestive tract.

The second abdominal branch of the vagus runs to the liver. Interestingly, these branches are closely linked to the feeling of hunger and desire for certain types of nutrients. The food we eat initially enters the stomach to be digested. Subsequently, they enter the small intestine, where most of our macronutrients (fats, carbohydrates, and protein amino acids) are absorbed into the bloodstream. These nutrients then penetrate the liver through the portal vein to be filtered and processed and send signals to the brain.

From the liver, the vagus transmits information to the brain about blood sugar level, fat intake, and general liver function. The vagus nerve can also transmit information about the amount of bile.

Necessary to help the digestion of fats. The liver performs numerous functions that require information transmitted by the vagus nerve, including but not limited to producing bile and bile salts (the active component of bile), which are then sent and stored in the gallbladder; balance blood sugar levels by producing glucose; control hunger and satiety by measuring fat intake; filter the blood in the portal vein, which carries all the nutrients and toxins from the intestine; and phase 1 and phase 2 of the detoxification processes of fat-soluble hormones, neurotransmitters, and toxins of the body. The liver is very important for our general well-being, and the innervation of the vagus is closely associated with maintaining this balance.

The gallbladder is intimately connected with the liver. Often overlooked by the medical system, the gallbladder is important for the optimal function of our body. When the liver creates bile and bile salts, they are sent to the gallbladder to be stored for the next meal. When the next meal occurs, the gallbladder pumps bile into the duodenum (the first part of the small intestine) to help incorporate fats into the bloodstream. This occurs in response to a meal that taste buds (sensory receptors in the tongue) determine that it contains fat, which must be digested when it reaches the small intestine.

The next branch of the bum is directed towards the pancreas. Your pancreas is one of the most important glands in the body, with an exocrine and endocrine component. The endocrine pancreas produces and secretes insulin and glucagon directly into the bloodstream to balance blood glucose levels (blood sugar). The exocrine pancreas produces and secretes digestive enzymes through a duct directly in the small intestine. The most important digestive enzymes produced by the pancreas are protease, which breaks down proteins into their amino acids; lipase, which breaks down the fats of its triglyceride components into free fatty acids and cholesterol; and amylase, which breaks down carbohydrates into simple sugars.

The innervation of the vagus sends signals from the pancreas to the brainstem, transmitting information about the status of exocrine and endocrine cells. It also transmits information from the brainstem to the organ about food intake and what enzymes are required for production and secretion in the bloodstream and digestive tract. The innervation of the vagus is essential to transmit information because of the lack of transmission of information alters the secretion of digestive enzymes, reducing the efficiency of the digestive process.

When the vagus nerve runs beyond the stomach, it forms the celiac plexus, consisting of a network formed between the sympathetic lumbar nerves and the parasympathetic fibers of the vagus. This network sends branches to the remaining organs in the abdomen.

The first innervated organ after the celiac plexus is the spleen. The spleen is located on the left side of your body, under the left lung, facing the liver. Its function is to monitor the bloodstream and activate or deactivate the cells of the immune system, depending on what it detects. During the first years of our life, both the spleen and the thymus control the function of immune cells, but later, when the thymus disappears, the system is controlled only by the spleen.

The spleen receives messages from the branches of the sympathetic system to activate the inflammatory pathways, which are activated in response to trauma or physical and biochemical damage. The parasympathetic branches send signals to stop the inflammation processes. The vagus nerve modulates a system called the anti-inflammatory cholinergic pathway, which has important effects on the spleen. In later sections, we will discuss these specific effects related to inflammation.

The next branch of the vagus after the celiac plexus extends into the small intestine. Once food has been degraded by chemical and physical agitation in the stomach, it penetrates the small intestine. Here they are subjected to another digestive process by pancreatic digestive enzymes and bile. The function of the small intestine is to degrade and absorb most of our macronutrients. These include fats, carbohydrates, and proteins (which must be degraded in their amino acid components). The bloodstream receives the macronutrients that have been accepted by the lining cells of the small intestine.

The bite of food we eat (which in this phase of the digestive process is called chyme) should be driven along the meandering course of the small intestine. For this to happen, the vagus nerve activates the smooth muscle cells of the digestive tract by transmitting information to the extensive network of nerves that line the intestine, called the enteric nervous system.

The small intestine is very long; it measures approximately 6.7 meters in length and is much longer than the next portion of the digestive tract: the large intestine.

We maintain a very important relationship with the other cells that inhabit our digestive tract. I mean the symbiotic relationship between our human cells and the bacteria that inhabit our intestines: our microbiome. The vast majority of our bacterial allies inhabit our large intestine, the thickest and shortest area of the digestive tract. Although these bacteria produce a large number of important vitamins, minerals, and biochemical precursors for us, they can also produce numerous toxins and gas. It is necessary that our system is able to keep these bacteria controlled and transmit signals to our brain about the status of the digestive tract and the function of the microbiome. Thus, although the vagus nerve activates smooth muscle cells to drive food through the rest of the digestive tract, it is also the main route of transmission for the microbiome to talk to the brain. The vagus nerve innervates approximately the first half of the large intestine: the ascending and transverse parts.

The last organ innervated by the vagus nerve actually consists of two organs, one located on each side of the body: the kidneys. These organs fulfill various functions that are crucial to our health. The kidneys remove fluid from the body in the form of urine, a combination of uric acid and water, which is then sent to the bladder. One of the main determinants of this control is blood pressure, which we will discuss in more detail in the next chapter. The vagus nerve is an important controller of kidney function, so it plays an important role in the control of blood pressure.

At the end of its path, the vagus nerve does not simply end but forms a final plexus with the parasympathetic nerves that run from the lower end of the spinal cord. These parasympathetic fibers innervate the second half of the large intestine, called the descending and sigmoid colon, as well as the bladder and sexual organs.

CORE FUNCTIONS OF THE VAGUS NERVE

An NV that works optimally is essential to optimize health and slow the development of diseases. There are numerous reasons for this, and in this chapter, we will review some of them.

A body that works at the optimum level is like a symphony orchestra. In a symphony, each of the various instruments plays a certain role, and optimal harmony can only be achieved if each instrument fulfills its mission. The conductor must ensure that no instrument is in tune or does not follow the tempo since a single mistake can ruin the performance. A director who does not fulfill his mission also leads to a dysfunctional performance.

The vagus nerve is the conductor of the symphony orchestra of the human body. It regulates the function of numerous organs and cells in our body, but it can only do so if it works optimally. You must be able to detect and transmit the appropriate information to the numerous organs and cells of the body. The dysfunctional transmission of information leads to a lack of harmony in the body, and eventually to a state of dysfunction and disease.

Let's analyze all the various functions that the orchestra director of the human body performs: the vagus nerve.

Feel the skin of the car

As we have commented in the previous chapter, the first branch of the vagus nerve is the atrial branch, which is specifically involved in feeling the skin of the atrium, the swallow, and the external ear canal of the ear.

The function of this branch consists purely of sensation, allowing us to feel pressure, touch, temperature, and humidity in the central section of each ear. Clinically, this is relevant and very important, since this is one of the main areas through which NV can be stimulated using techniques such as acupuncture.

Allow you to swallow food

When we eat, we can't think of the process of swallowing each bite and stop the reflex of breathing so as not to choke. This important task is controlled by the vagus nerve.

The second branch of the NV (the pharyngeal branch) controls the activation of five muscles of the pharynx: the three constrictor muscles located at the back of the throat and two other muscles that connect the throat and the soft palate (the soft tissue in the back of the palate). These muscles are involved in the pharyngeal phase of swallowing, which involves causing the chewed food to descend into the larynx and esophagus, preventing it from entering the trachea, keeping the airway clear. This branch of the NV also controls the active motor component of the gag reflex.

Clinically this is important since a bad function of the vagus nerve causes cough and a change in the function of the gag reflex. We can use this reflex to help tone the NV with active exercises and activating the gag reflex.

Control your airways and vocal cords

Every time you breathe, are you aware of the effort needed to keep your upper airways open? The muscles that participate in this process also participate in the production of your voice. If you've ever wondered which nerve makes it possible for you to communicate verbally with those around you, the answer is simple: it's the vague nerve!

The third and fourth branches of the NV are the superior and recurrent laryngeal nerves. The upper laryngeal branch is responsible for the muscles located on the vocal cords, while the recurrent laryngeal branch is responsible for the muscles located under the strings.

The upper laryngeal branch transmits motor information to some muscles of the larynx and controls the vocal tone. A bad function of the upper laryngeal branch causes a change in the tone of voice. A chronically hoarse voice or a monotonous voice that gets tired easily is a symptom of a low vagal tone (ability to transmit information) in this branch of the nerve. Irritation of this nerve can also cause a severe cough and risk of aspiration (food or drink that enters the trachea due to poor vocal cord function).

The recurrent laryngeal branch transmits motor information to the muscles under the vocal cords, allowing sounds to be formed by opening, closing, and tensing the vocal cord structures. It also has a sensory component that transmits information of the esophagus, trachea, and internal mucous membranes of these structures. Dysfunction of these nerves leads to hoarseness, loss of voice, and respiratory problems during physical activity.

These laryngeal muscles control the opening, closing, and function of the airways. Therefore, any difficulty in breathing or speaking can be attributed to poor function and tone of the vagus nerve. Breathing and muscle tone of the airways are extremely important for vagal function. Any chronic obstruction that prevents the airways from being clear and functioning correctly affects the function and transmission of information of these muscles, negatively affecting the function of your vagus nerve.

Control breathing

And the breath? Well, the bum also plays a role in controlling this important function. Pulmonary branch

The NV runs to the pulmonary plexus, connects with the sympathetic nervous system, and innervates the trachea and bronchi of both lungs. The vague component is a sensory nerve that transmits information to the brain about lung expansion levels, as well as oxygen and carbon dioxide levels.

In the lungs, activation of the vagus nerve slows the respiratory rate and makes breathing deeper. During the rest-and-digestion phase, breathing tends to be deeper and comes from the diaphragm instead of accessory muscles for breathing, and the respiratory rate tends to be lower. When a person passes from the fight-or-flight state to the rest-and-digestion phase, slow and deep breathing activates the vagus nerve and stimulates the relaxation reflex.

It is necessary that the tone of the vagus nerve is optimal to open the airways in the pharynx, larynx, and trachea. The muscles of the pharynx and larynx are innervated by the motor components of the NV. The poor activity of these neurons can cause airway obstruction, as occurs in chronic obstructive pulmonary disease (COPD) and obstructive sleep apnea. Both disorders are a sign of a low vagal tone and that it is necessary to activate the nerve. I even dare to say that the obstruction of these airways can be the main cause of vagus nerve dysfunction, in which we will abound in more detail in later chapters.

Control heart rate

Your heart beats to transport blood containing nutrients and oxygen to each of your cells, and transport toxins to the organs capable of eliminating them. The NV plays a prominent role in making heart rate.

Stay within acceptable levels when the body is not stressed. Without the NV, our heart would not work near its optimal frequency.

The vagus nerve is connected to the sinoatrial nodule, which sends electrical signals to the two atria (the thin cavities in the upper part of the heart). It is also directly connected to the atrioventricular nodule, which controls the pumping frequency and contraction pressure of the ventricles (the two lower, thicker cavities of the heart).

During moments of fight-or-flight, the sympathetic nervous system activates the heart to increase the frequency of pumping and the pressure of contractions in the two ventricles. When the stressor has passed, the resting-and-digestion phase is imposed, and the body enters the vagal activation phase. At this time, the parasympathetic fibers of the NV slow down the heart rate and actively reduce the pressure of the pumping contractions. These fibers work to reduce the activity of the heart, allowing it to rest and recover from moments of stress and strong activation.

Maintain optimal blood pressure

Blood pressure is a determining factor in the amount of fluid present in the bloodstream. The kidneys work to filter and eliminate fluids and toxins from the body, and are, therefore, the main controllers of blood pressure in the body. The vagus nerve transmits information to and from the kidneys to help them control the flow of water and fluid within the renal glomeruli, the basic filtering unit of the kidneys, thus controlling the general blood pressure of the body.

When the body is under stress, the blood vessels (specifically the carotid body) transmit ascending signals to the brainstem and descending to the kidneys through the vagus and sympathetic nerves. Next, the kidneys contract their blood vessels and increase blood pressure by reducing the amount of water they filter and remove from the bloodstream. When the body is relaxed, the signals transmitted by the carotid body order the kidneys to remove more water and dilate the blood vessels to lower blood pressure.

The hormones are also intimately connected with this process, collaborating with the vagus and sympathetic nerves. However, immediate control comes from nerves, while slow and progressive control is determined by hormones.

Hypertension is a very common diagnosis, and, frequently, the doctor prescribes a medication to control these levels. Hypertension may be a sign of overactivation of the stress hormones of the adrenal glands, and the response to stress, which occurs through the sympathetic nerves. It is also a very common sign of vagus nerve dysfunction and low vagal tone.

Control the numerous functions of the liver

The vagus nerve transmits important information to and from the liver, controlling almost 500 tasks. In this section, I will discuss only some of the best-known functions.

The liver regulates where blood flows in the body. In times of stress, when the body enters a fight-or-flight state, blood flow is propelled to the arms and legs to increase muscle activation and allow us to defend ourselves from an attack or escape from it. Blood flow in the liver is reduced since digestion, and blood filtration during this stressful event is not a priority for survival. When the body is relaxed, and at rest-and-digestion phase, activation of the vagus nerve increases, and blood flow to the liver increases as well. During these moments, digestion, blood filtering, and other functions are prioritized to optimize cell status.

The vagus nerve also controls the liver cells that are responsible for producing bile and bile salts, as well as transporting bile to the gallbladder and small intestine. It is shown that, when the vagus nerve is active, these cells, called cholangiocytes, are active and increase the flow of bile into the gallbladder for storage.

Bile performs multiple functions for the liver and body. The liver detoxifies fat-soluble toxins through a two-phase process, creating water-soluble residues that must be eliminated. Bile contains these toxins that have become harmless and are prepared to be eliminated from the body through the digestive tract through our feces. The stool is one of the three routes through which we eliminate waste. The other methods of waste disposal are urine through the kidneys or sweat through the skin.

Bile salts, the effective component of bile, play another role. When bile is released in the small intestine, waste and bile salts are released. Bile salts have to escort triglycerides (fat molecules) from the digestive tract, through the enterocytes (the cells that line the small intestine), until they are absorbed into the bloodstream. If they are not escorted by bile salts, fats cannot be absorbed, which is very harmful, since fats and cholesterol perform numerous vital functions in the body.

The vagus nerve is the tenth of the twelve cranial nerves and is the longest in the body. In fact, the word vagus means "wanderer" in Latin, which perfectly illustrates the path of this nerve that extends through various organs of the body.

The vagus nerve is born in the cranial box, exactly in the medulla, and descends through the neck, developing into two branches that reach the abdomen through the different organs that it finds along the way.

The vagus nerve intervenes in the sensitivity of the respiratory mucous membranes and transmits the rhythm, strength, and frequency of breathing. It innervates the pharynx, larynx, esophagus, trachea, and bronchi, in addition to supplying nerve fibers to the heart, stomach, pancreas, and liver. However, it also handles the reverse mission; that is, it receives the signals from the internal organs and sends them to the brain for processing.

Although perhaps the most interesting is the relationship between the vagus nerve and anxiety since it also transmits the signs of nervousness or calm, anger, or relaxation.

The sympathetic nervous system prepares us for action, so it feeds primarily on hormones such as adrenaline and cortisol. The parasympathetic nervous system is involved in rest and relaxation.

In practice, both systems function as an accelerator and decelerator. The sympathetic nervous system accelerates and activates us while the parasympathetic nervous system helps us relax and reduce speed, for which it uses neurotransmitters such as acetylcholine, which decreases heart rate and blood pressure to make organs function more slowly.

The ventral vagal system

The ventral vagal system of social engagement, which is in action when we are at rest, or at least when we are not threatened, helps us to engage with the environment, with others, and with ourselves.

It also helps us to regulate the sympathetic-adrenal system and keeps us in a tolerance window, which is very important when working on trauma.

When we are threatened, however, the ventral vagal system is overridden by the sympathetic system (Porges calls this the sympathetic-adrenal), which mobilizes the combat survival and flight response. The tonsil sets off the alarm signal, and the hypothalamus sets off a cascade of substances, which include cortisol, epinephrine, adrenaline, and others, to mobilize our energy against the threat.

Activation of the sympathetic system, therefore, results in an increased flow of blood to the muscles of the body, giving them more energy to fight or flee. The flow to the cerebral cortex is then decreased, so we don't think as well, as part of the brain is turned off. It increases our vigilance. All of these reactions optimize our chances of survival.

VAGUS NERVE AND ENERGY PSYCHOLOGY

Often, however, the ventral vagal system of engagement and the fight/flight response are not proportional to the threat. In this case, the dorsal vagal system activates automatically. It is the most primitive system, and it is triggered by a lack of oxygen in the tissues and muscles. In other words, when we run out of fuel for movement, to defend ourselves or to flee, then it pushes the brain to put itself in a position of immobility.

We see this in the animal world when mammals simulate death. The typical example is that of immobilizing yourself like an opossum.

The immobility reaction that starts when the dorsal vagal system blocks many bodily functions leads to a reduction in heart rate and breathing and is accompanied by numbness.

While this stillness protects our survival, if active for a long time, it can be absolutely fatal; people can die from it (leading to heart and respiratory problems, among many other disorders).

The nerve of the vagal system has two main branches that meet where the heart branch is connected. The heart is very important in terms of polyvagal science, and this is also where energy psychology meets polyvagal science.

Almost every organ system in the body is affected by the vagal nerve, also called the vagus nerve, which is the longest nerve in the body. It starts at the tenth cranial nerve and threads through the spinal cord and the spine, then it connects to all these different organ systems: the lungs, the heart, the stomach, the spleen, the liver, the colon, kidney, small intestine, etc.

Porges considers the autonomic nervous system from the point of view of safety, an important subject when working with trauma. When we are in a safe place, we have optimal activation, we are at rest, and we digest, we are connected to the ventral vagal system - the engagement system -, and we notice and participate in visual contact, facial expression, vocalization, and other social behaviors. When the danger appears, we begin to go into hyperactivation mode. Our heart rate accelerates, the sympathetic system, the adrenal system start, we mobilize the energy of the fight / flee response and survive. You can also experience dissociated rabies and panic.

When we go to the level of threat to life (when our organism perceives that we are going to die), we change. Instead of hyperactivation, we are hypoactivation. We descend into the dorsal vagal branch of the parasympathetic system, and we have a very low heart rate. With some people, the heart stops during this change. We pass in stillness instead of mobility; it's blocking. We undergo a dissociated collapse.

When we visualize the polyvagal system by looking from the top to the bottom of the organism, we see a ladder of nerve fibers that goes from the brain to the heart. It's not just the blood flow, but electromagnetic energy which is very important for understanding energy psychology.

Porges suggests that when we feel safe with others, we can then communicate with other people. This is where we can make eye contact, smile, listen, and we have what he calls prosody, a certain rhythm and intonation, which is very pleasant and a tone higher than grave in the voice. The first step in a relationship or engagement is to help the other person feel safe. Of course, you have to help yourself to feel safe. Safety is really fundamental, and it comes from the ventral vagal system.

The parasympathetic nervous system on the vagal nerve is different in the states of danger and threat: a distinction is made between the recovery parasympathetic and the immobilized, dissociated parasympathetic. When we sense the danger, the old vagal system (back) increases its activity. When we are challenged, we try to speak first, to negotiate if possible; then we go into fight/flight, then we block. The only exception to this is in situations where the ventral vagal is completely passed. This can happen for a variety of reasons, such as with pain patients who are exhausting people who are helping them to take care of themselves. As people withdraw or judge them, they have learned not to communicate. They go even more than in this blocking state. Often also when we are in combat mode, if we cannot respond to the threat, we will automatically go into the dorsal vagal blockade.

Energy psychology articulates with the polyvagal system in several interesting ways that have health care implications for all of us. Energy psychology brings together a family of integrative approaches to care, which is organized around three major elements of the energy system: the bioenergetic field around the body, the chakras as energy centers, and the meridian system in the form of energy trajectories, which runs all over the body with acupoints, which can be stimulated to create various reactions.

For example, some people work on tranquilizers and others on energizers. To make the link with the polyvagal system, if you have a very active client, you will seek to know more about the tranquilizing points as shown by Donna Eden's work on energy medicine, of course, you find the points that are most stimulating for people who are depressed, more closed, more blocked.

Energy psychology also joins the polyvagal system at the level of the heart. The heart has its own nervous system, which we can think of as a kind of brain. What we know from research by the Institute is that the energy field of the heart is more powerful than the energy field of the brain (about 100,000 times more powerful than the electric field of the brain and up to 5,000 times more powerful than the magnetic field of the brain).

Researchers have also shown that the heart's brain exists. In other words, the heart has its own nervous system, which we can think of as a kind of brain. It turns out that the heart initiates more messages to the brain than the brain does to the heart. What this means is that it is our engagement with ourselves and with those at very in a loving and reassuring way, which makes us want these signals to be sent to the brain. We want it to inform our thinking, our plans, and our decisions in life, and now we know that anatomy supports this idea.

The importance of heart variability

The autonomic nervous system is very important because it regulates everything automatically, and we need to know how the body does this.

There are many ways to find out, but one way is called heart variability. It is measured in the interval between heartbeats.

The autonomic nervous system plays an immense role in cardiac variability. If a person is depressed or has low variability, it means that their heart is beating too regularly. This reflects the reduced ability of the autonomic nervous system to regulate everything in order to remain healthy: homeostasis, the ability to manage internal and external aggressive factors, threats, etc. Every day we face threats of one kind or another (relationship threats, threats from our own body because we have a disease, an autoimmune condition, or whatever you want). Cardiac variability measures the ability to regulate and recover from internal and external aggressive factors.

In addition to measuring the regulatory functioning of the autonomic nervous system, cardiac variability is also an index of regulated emotional reactions. We look for coherence, and energetic psychology, we talk a lot about coherence. When people use energy healing methods, whether it's Energy Psychology or Energy Medicine, what really interests us is this idea of coherence - the integrative, cognitive, and emotional states where you feel calm and focused. It's a consistency of all these different systems. When you are in this position where the systems are synchronized with each other, and there is a harmony between all these processes: thought, emotional, physiological, etc. then we have health. You are centered in a position where you can think more clearly.

Simple tools like cardiac breathing (where you imagine feeling inhaling in the heart and exhaling through the heart) help people create calm and inner balance. Research has been able to measure all kinds of great results with this practice. Increased heart variability is one of them, which means great flexibility, as well as hope, self-esteem, self-efficacy, and certainly mental, emotional, and physiological health. So this is a very important approach.

In terms of stress management and the consequences of trauma, energy treatments transmitted at a distance, therefore without direct contact with a therapist, are particularly effective because they work at your own pace so that you can find certain well-being in your daily life.

Roger Callahan and the variability of the heart rate

Roger Callahan, who developed mental field therapy (TFT - the precursor to EFT), has performed a large number of experiments where he has shown that cardiac variability improves after treatment for TFT.

The central problem with that, and their research, is that we lack randomized controlled trials. "What I would say is that we already know in energy psychology that we need to improve our research, randomization, controlled studies, etc. ; so it's not new. But I think we can't ignore some of the Callahan data, "says Maggie Philipps.

One of his reports deals with 20 cases of people with diagnoses of heart problems (i.e., very low heart variability, very rigid heart rhythms, and it is not good for health, or the rest). After a brief intervention with TFT, which involves stimulating a prescribed sequence of meridian points, he found a huge improvement, large increases in heart variability.

Today we need more randomized controlled studies that link the results to variability in heart rate. The CAPE research committee is actively involved in this area, and there are more and more good studies coming out. We also need to teach heart rate variability more widely in order to provide protocols and develop instruments that are simple and affordable, and then, of course, link that to research that actually proves it to be effective.

HRV is a measure of the health of the polyvagal system. One of the reasons why energy psychology is so effective is that we are working on this non-verbal vagal system. Stephen Porges was the first to quantify and use VFC in psychophysiological research. What really puzzled Porges was what is known as the "polyvagal paradox." There are these mechanisms that mediate certain aspects of our stress response, etc., but can we explain how they mediate respiratory sinus arrhythmia, which is a protective measure, and bradycardia, which is fatal? The vagal production of a branch towards the heart is linked to the myelinated vagal system, which promotes calm, relaxation and inhibits the activation of the fight or flees response and the hypothalamic-pituitary-adrenal (HHS) axis.

The other branch, or other types of vagal system, the non-myelinated vagus nerve, which is connected to both the sympathetic-adrenal circuit and the dorsal vagal circuit, is manifest in bradycardia; it's the fatal heart reaction. The two together form, in fact, cardiac respiration.

Porges is now working on developing ways to identify and measure heart rhythms specifically related to these two different types of vagal circuits because we need to understand them both. We need to understand what is causing the change in this wonderful positive state of calm and relaxation in hell.

So trauma inhibits the vagal braking system and compromises the ability to regulate affections and emotions. One of the basic ways in which we use energy medicine, energy healing, energy psychology, at least emotionally, is when people are upset. Again, the more we work with, the more we treat this vagal brake system, the faster the person can recover and calm down emotionally, which of course, leads to all kinds of health issues.

CHAPTER FIVE
HOW TO OVERCOME A TRAUMA

It has long been thought that the symptoms of trauma were the result of the type and intensity of an external event. While the magnitude of the stressor is clearly important, it does not define trauma. This is because the trauma is not in the event itself, but that it resides in the nervous system. Trauma related to a single event (unlike prolonged neglect and abuse) is physiological, not psychological.

What is trauma? Why, after a traumatic experience, does one become hypervigilant, frightened, aggressive? Why do we have nightmares, flashbacks, and uncontrollable fears?

All this can be explained by the activity of the Autonomous Nervous System (ANS). Polyvagal Theory sheds new light on how the ANS works, from trauma to social behavior.

The absolute goal of the autonomic nervous system is to keep us alive

The ANS is a kind of automatic pilot of the human body, which allows the heart to beat, the lungs to breathe, or the digestive system to do its job automatically, without us having to at any time need it to think for it to happen.

Its role also lies in permanent monitoring of our environment: it continually scans the external and internal world of the individual, always on guard, in order to check if we are safe. This process is completely beyond conscious awareness: Stephen Porges suggests the term "neuroception" describe how the nervous system detects danger and safety signals in the environment, without the conscious parts of the brain being involved.

Conventionally, it has long been considered that only two opposite modes of the nervous system, made up of two distinct branches, were involved in the functioning of the body. The polyvagal theory offers a different understanding, comprising three branches:

the parasympathetic nervous system made up of the vagus nerve, which starts from the brainstem and innervates many organs. It separates itself into two branches:

the ventral vagal tract, which is linked to the feeling of security and social bond: when you feel good, relaxed and open to social relationships, it is this path that is connected

the dorsal vagal pathway, which response to signals of extreme danger with a collapse response and disconnects from the relational bond: when one feels paralyzed, numb or absent, it is this pathway that is connected

the sympathetic nervous system, located in the central part of the spinal cord, which prepares for action: its activation allows the release of adrenaline and triggers the "Fight or Flight" defense system.

Polyvagal theory

We can represent these three branches of the nervous system as a hierarchical scale of the stress response: at the top is the "green zone," in which we feel relaxed, open to conversation, and the exchange of points of view. In the two lower floors, the connection capacity is replaced by protection mechanisms: in the yellow zone, strong energy is mobilized to defend itself, and going down again, we arrive at the "red zone" in which the system is placed Standby.

Safety Polyvagal

- Heartbeats slowly, breathing is regulated
- Saliva and digestion are stimulated
- Facial muscles are activated (emotions, facial expressions
- Increased prosody and eye contact
- Good connection to the human voice
- Good connection to the world and to people, ability to play

- Efficient immune system
- General well-being (sleep, health, digestion, blood pressure.

Polyvagal danger

- Accelerated heart rate, short, shallow breath
- Increase in pain tolerance
- Little facial expression

When the ANS detects danger, the hearing system changes: less listening to the human voice, the muscles of the middle ear are more connected with high and low frequencies (which correspond to predator frequencies).

Anxiety, anxiety attacks, anger, difficulty concentrating and doing things right, relationship problems

Heart disease, high cholesterol, anxiety disorders, digestive & sleep problems, weight gain, headache, poor immune system

Freeze Polyvagal

When there is no possibility of running away or fighting in the face of life threatening danger, the nervous system freezes

- Stillness response
- Reduction in blood flow, especially to the brain
- Preparing for death when no other option is available
- No feeling or emotion
- Chronic fatigue, dissociation, depression, fibromyalgia, low blood pressure

FREEZING AND TRAUMA

Healthy people can move from the "green area" to the "yellow area" easily and flexibly, as shown in the following example:

I'm on the terrace of a restaurant with friends; I'm at ease in conversation, I eat with pleasure and enjoy this moment of relaxation (green zone).

Suddenly, I see a big dog running towards me running at top speed. I instantly grab a chair nearby to block the animal (yellow area). His guard whistles to call him close to him. The dog immediately obeys, and I return to a state of relaxation (green zone) after a few moments, once the possible danger has been averted.

When Combat or Flight is not an option, the nervous system "chooses" the Freeze. The reaction of the nervous system does not depend on what one thinks is the right way to react to a danger, the ANS imposes its response automatically, according to its reading of the situation. So when the fear is really too great, and the nervous system sees no other way out, the system goes to sleep.

This phenomenon of paralysis of the organism can often be understood to be the cause of many symptoms or anxiety states such as panic attacks, OCD, phobias, etc.

In addition, many disorders and pathologies (depression, schizophrenia, borderline personality, the spectrum of autism) are affected by dysregulation of the nervous system, some of the manifestations of which are very similar to those observed in trauma:

- Difficulty feeling safe
- Hearing hypersensitivity
- Little facial expression
- Lack of prosody (you're monotonous)

When under stress, let the nervous system complete its "activation cycle."

As in the example of the little fawn and its mother in the video above, a very frightening and hopeless situation can give rise to a state of freezing, the response of the dorsal vagal nerve. Here, the driver of the car turns off the engine to remove the source of stress, without any further action on its part. The fawn mom can gently reassure her little one, she simply manifests her presence with the right distance, without intrusion, leaving the nervous system all the space and time it needs to return to the "green zone."

In humans, the activation cycle does not end as quickly as in animals, but the principle is the same. The reassuring and non-invasive presence of a caring person allows the nervous system to calm down.

Returning to the "green zone" is crucial for the health

It is essential to feel safe in order to be able to live fully and in good health. When this is the case, the brain releases oxytocin; we have better learning and production capacities, we are more relaxed and pleasant; we are loved by others, the organs work better ...

In order to help the nervous system go up the ladder, it is useful to focus on a few practices:

- slow breathing, with a longer exhalation than inspiration
- speak with a smile and look in the eyes
- sing, solo or better, in a choir
- evolve in an environment that seems safe
- avoid complicated relationships, which reinforce insecurity
- practice a wind instrument
- listen to music, preferably female voices

CHAPTER SIX.
CHIROPRACTIC ACTION

WHAT IS CHIROPRACTIC

Chiropractic is a safe option to create more health in your life. It is the science that specializes in the spine and nervous system.

The central nervous system is made up of the brain and its continuation, the spinal cord. From the spinal cord, and through the vertebrae, all nerve endings go out to our entire body: organs, tissues, muscles, etc. The nervous system is the head of our body and, with a nervous system functioning and yielding 100%, our entire body works better.

There are internal forces that work permanently for the creation and maintenance of our bodies. When the internal communication of the body begins to fail, these internal forces take time to manifest themselves and begin the inconsistencies that later lead to symptoms and diseases.

Chiropractic helps protect and restore internal communication, even before symptoms are perceived. Chiropractic care throughout life and early correction facilitate the maintenance of health.

The word chiropractic comes from the Greek and means 'manual practice'. It is based on the principle that healing of the body can only be completed when the skeletal system is functioning optimally, which happens by having properly aligned vertebrae.

To do this, the chiropractor uses their hands or an instrument called 'activator' to make adjustments; the specific manipulations of the vertebrae.

When the bones of the spine do not articulate correctly, a condition known as vertebral subluxation occurs; Neural transmission is disturbed and causes dysfunction in the back, as well as in other regions of the body.

These exercises will teach us how to combat anxiety. ISR exercises are a series of simple exercises that, once learned, can be worked at home and are designed to offer a new adaptation of the body and facilitate personal healing. These exercises will teach us how to combat anxiety:

Teach listening to body rhythms and inner wisdom through consciousness, breathing, movement, and touch.

We use new breathing, movement, and attention patterns to reconnect the body and mind safely. The body then leaves its state of defense and moves towards growth, well-being, vitality, the desire to participate fully in life, and maintain an internal state of harmony.

The combination of these exercises with any other chiropractic technique allows for deeper and more sustainable results.

At the Allard Chiropractic Center, we give you the tools to adapt your body and mind to the environment and reduce anxiety.

Anxiety and stress are the way we have adapted physiologically to events.

Same situation

Depending on the state of preception in which you are, it can vary, and it goes from being a threat to a calm and safe situation.

The physiology of stress

It occurs when the number of messages received per second has overwhelmed the brain due to a physical, chemical, or emotional stimulus. Then the body and mind are disconnected, and the spine assumes a defensive posture.

This dangerous perception

it is stored in the body in the form of tension, and over time it manifests itself in muscular contractures, spinal distortion, reduced breathing of the affected area, limitation of movement and discomfort, or nervousness.

In an attitude of defense

The blood supply of the neocortex is diminished, and the signals are diverted to the most primitive and reactive part of the brain, causing more stiffness, higher blood pressure, and the reaction to new stresses will increase.

So stress is a perception of our body and mind to defend against danger. So to start knowing how to combat anxiety, we would have to ask ourselves the following question: Is stress desirable?

We do not treat all patients with the same technique or frequency, depending on the person we use more mechanical techniques or others that work with internal tension.

Once the course of visits is determined, the chiropractor can use different techniques:

Is stress normal?

↑ YES

Momentary stress is a natural and healthy physiological reaction that allows the body to respond to a specific dangerous situation.

↓ NO

Sustained stress is a pattern of tension due to an unnatural perception of being in a situation of permanent danger.

We do not intend to combat anxiety from a medical point of view or as a disease.

What is intended is to give the individual the possibility to control and regulate their own physiology through consciousness.

Sometimes we have the feeling that stress follows us wherever we go. It seems that the path we take or the work we do or how old we are is not the same.

There are countless studies that demonstrate the adverse effects of excess stress on our health.

But do we really need articles to affirm that excess stress is not good for our body and makes us feel horrible? It seems that if.

And it is only when we reach the limit and we can no longer, that we start looking for solutions and there are still many people who still do not think about resorting to chiropractic care to overcome it.

But first, it is important to understand how the body reacts to stress. There are basic "channels" through which we perceive stress: Environment, body, and emotions.

Environmental stress: Let's say you are walking along a quiet road and hear a loud bang near you, similar to an explosion. That is environmental stress. Pollution would be another example. Over this stress, we have no control.

Body stress: includes diseases, lack of sleep, poor nutrition, lack of hydration.

Emotional stress: it is slightly different because it is based on how we interpret certain things

The type of stress we can handle the most is emotional stress, it is the only one we have control over, and it is also the one that affects us the most.

Did you know that even children suffer stress?

According to a large study by the American Psychological Association (APA), almost a third of the children surveyed indicated that they had experienced physical symptoms associated with stress in the month prior to the study, for example, problems falling asleep, stomach aches, and Headaches. And even more amazing, the rate of youth suicides today is four times higher than in the 1950s.

In this modern society, we are overstressed. Over the years, many studies have been carried out to assess the impact of chronic stress on the body and its consequences, such as these common symptoms: feeling irritable, angry, overwhelmed, anxious, fatigued, and depressed.

What happens to the body when we suffer stress? What areas are affected?

The musculoskeletal system: the muscles tense and contract, causing headaches, migraines, and other conditions.

The respiratory: high stress can cause rapid breathing or hyperventilation and trigger panic or anxiety attacks.

Cardiovascular system: acute stress can accelerate heart rate and inflammation in the coronary arteries, which can increase the risk of stroke,

And the nervous system: the body will act as if it were under threat. This reaction is an innate response that has been going on for millions of years and has allowed human beings to survive. When the mind perceives a threat or the body experiences a shock, our body releases hormones that increase the ability to fight or flee

Regardless of the cause, if a fight/flight response is initiated, it not only affects an area of the body but also triggers the nervous system that is the base or root of our entire organism, so it ends up affecting our entire body... It would be like this:

The brain awakens the sympathetic nervous system and increases heart rate, blood volume, and blood pressure. This diverts blood from the digestive system and extremities. The adrenal glands also emit a cocktail of chemicals, including adrenaline, epinephrine, and norepinephrine, which can wreak havoc on a person's health over time.

Persistent tension causes the muscles to contract and the spine to be locked in an "abnormal" position, which in turn interferes with the optimal functioning of the nervous system. Consequently, it can affect the body's immune response and delay general healing.

By working on the spine, the base from which tension impulses radiate throughout the body, the chiropractor can help patients cope better with stress.

The chiropractor will put the spine in place because if it is misaligned, the nervous system cannot correctly send messages through the body. Better vertebral alignment will mean better communication and greater system efficiency. Chiropractic adjustments will release muscle tension, calm irritated nerves.

CHIROPRACTIC CORRECTION

Chiropractic correction is a procedure in which trained specialists (chiropractors) use their hands or a small instrument to apply a rapid and controlled force to a spinal joint. The purpose of this procedure, also known as spinal manipulation, is to improve the movement of the spine and improve the physical function of the body.

Why is it done?

Low back, neck, and head pain are the three most common problems for which people request a chiropractic adjustment.

Request a consultation at Mayo Clinic

Risks

Chiropractic correction is safe when performed by a trained and licensed person to provide chiropractic care. Serious complications related to chiropractic correction are, in general, rare, but may include the following:

- A herniated disc or a worsening of an existing herniated disc
- Compression of nerves in the lower spine (horsetail syndrome)
- A certain type of stroke (dissection of the vertebral artery) after neck manipulation

Don't try to undergo a chiropractic correction if you have the following:

- Severe osteoporosis
- Numbness, tingling or loss of strength in an arm or leg
- Spinal cancer
- An increased risk of stroke
- A known bone abnormality in the upper neck

Chiropractic treatment may require a series of sessions with a chiropractor, but most people achieve maximum improvement in 10 sessions. Many health insurance policies cover chiropractic care, but you could confirm how many treatments are covered within a certain period.

What you can expect

At the first consultation, the chiropractor will ask you questions about your medical history and perform a physical exam with special attention to the spine. You may also recommend that you have other tests or studies, such as an x-ray.

During the procedure

During a typical chiropractic correction, the chiropractor puts you in specific positions to treat the affected areas. Often, you lie on your stomach on a padded chiropractic stretcher with a specific design. The chiropractor applies force suddenly and controlled with the hands in a joint to push it out of its usual range of motion. You may hear clicks or cracks while the chiropractor moves the joints in the treatment session.

After the procedure

Some people experience minor side effects for a few days after chiropractic correction. These may include headache, fatigue, or pain in the parts of the body that were treated.

Chiropractic adjustment can be effective in treating lower back pain, although much of the research done reveals only a modest benefit, similar to the results of more conventional treatments. Some studies suggest that spinal manipulation may also be effective for headaches and other disorders related to the spine, such as neck pain.

Not all people respond to chiropractic adjustments. A lot depends on your particular situation. If the symptoms do not begin to improve after several weeks of treatment, chiropractic adjustment may not be the best option for you.

CHAPTER SEVEN

VAGUS NERVE AND ANXIETY: EXERCISES TO TONE AND REDUCE STRESS

The vagus nerve is one of those responsible for relaxing your body. Among its functions is to reduce the heart rate, relax your breathing, improve your digestion, among other things. The good news that I want to share with you is that it is in your hands to be able to make your vagus nerve healthy and strong so that it can fulfill this function of relaxing your body every time you need it.

The vagus nerve activates your parasympathetic system

The vagus nerve is a very important component of our body, for this reason, I recommend you to get to know and recognize it because through it you can even know how to help your body to reactivate its functions of the parasympathetic system (which is what relaxes us and restore) and thus maintain your balance.

As on other occasions, I have told you, your nervous system is responsible for regulating virtually all the sensations involved in stress and anxiety. The nervous system starts from your brain, sending signals to the different parts of your body that perform functions automatically, including your heartbeat, breathing, digestion, and so on. It is also up to the nervous system to activate your body when faced with stressful situations, as well as relax it once the dangerous situation has passed. To relax, we will need to activate our parasympathetic system, and it turns out that most of the functions that are performed during this activation are performed by your vagus nerve.

The vague nerve "wanders" throughout your body and is the longest of all

From your head, specifically from the brain, 12 pairs of cranial nerves, which will go to the rest of your body to transmit or receive different information, is the way we have to connect brain to body. And the tenth of these cranial nerves is the vagus nerve.

They are said to be cranial nerves because it is divided into two, the right and left vagus nerve, and between them, they are responsible for 75% of functions of the parasympathetic system. In other words, it is the vagus nerve that is responsible for relaxing.

Your vagus nerve is the longest of all cranial nerves and travels your body practically from the anus to your brain. And from my point of view, we are most interested in learning in relation to stress and anxiety.

Among the multiple functions of the vagus nerve, we find the following:

- Regulates the motor functions of the larynx, diaphragm, stomach, and heart.
- It generates the sensory functions of the tongue, ears and visceral organs (stomach, intestine, kidneys, and liver)

In other words, it is in charge of reducing the intensity of your heart rate, calming your breathing, regulating your digestion, expressing sensations of your throat, tongue, and ear, regulating the activity of the kidneys and liver, thus helping to improve your immune system too.

As you can see, there are too many functions in which the vagus nerve is involved; it also performs motor functions, that means that it gives movement to certain parts of the body, and on the other hand, it makes you aware of the different sensations you have in your body.

Fun fact: humming or cooing activates the vague nerve of the mother who practices it and, at the same time, helps activate and relax your child's.

How do I know that I need to tone my vagus nerve?

If you perceive any of the following sensations, it will be of great benefit to pay attention to your vagus nerve:

- Rare sensations in the tongue

- Difficulty to swallow
- Feeling of having something stuck in the throat
- Irregularities in your digestion
- Sudden changes in your heart rate
- Difficulty tasting food
- Tension in the muscles of your face
- Feeling of not being able to talk when you feel stressed
- Sudden onset of nausea
- Difficulty feeling connected to other people
- Excess empathy or affection for bad news
- Difficulty to socialize

You may also have rare sensations in the ear, so giving tone to the vagus nerve can also help reduce tinnitus.

VAGUE NERVE, EMPATHY, AND SOCIALIZATION

Something interesting about the vagus nerve is that it is also stimulated through socialization. Many of its functions have to do with regulating facial expressions and the tone of your voice, that is why the way you feel can be reflected in how you are speaking and in the expressions of your face, thus sending a message to the other about your current state.

It is also involved in generating oxytocin, which is the attachment hormone, which we secrete from when we are breastfeeding until when we have sex. That is why positive socialization and connection ties with other people, will help lower stress levels, and it is scientifically proven that it also prevents degenerative neuronal diseases.

At the same time, the vagus nerve is activated when we are facing another person, and we need to regulate facial expressions. That is why, one way to stimulate our vagus nerve is through specific facial movements, in addition to a healthy socialization.

Do you have trouble talking or opening up with other people when you feel bad?

When we have a history that has caused post-traumatic stress, we probably also have the need to work with our vagus nerve, because precisely a feature that arises after having experienced trauma experiences, is the difficulty of speaking or approaching other people in times of stress emotional. At the same time, you are likely to feel an excess of empathy in relation to the problems of others, all this has to do with the same, and stimulating your vagus nerve can help you.

Many times we disconnect to protect ourselves, avoid socialization so as not to feel in danger, but if we learn to give a positive tone to our vagus nerve, it can even help us to feel connected to others in a healthy and positive way.

Some scientists also link the vagus nerve with feelings such as gratitude and compassion for oneself and others.

SO HOW TO TONE OUR VAGUS NERVE

So, until now, we have understood that the need to give tone to our vagus nerve is born that the better it is, the better our ability to relax, that is, the easier and faster we can get to do it.

There are many things we can do to tone our vague nerve, what I recommend is that you do not abuse them, or do them with the intention of "urging me to relax my body." Remember that the intention is to offer help to your body, but with love and living it with awareness.

Wash your face with cold water - bath with fresh water

Instinctively when we feel bad, we go to the bathroom to wet our faces, right? Well, it is precisely because the freshwater on the face, forehead, and neck, will help tone your vagus nerve. Hence also that baths with fresh water are recommended.

Sings

Has it happened to you, or do you know someone who, after taking singing lessons, changed his life in many ways? As it turns out, singing will also tone your vague nerve, so put your favorite songs and sing.

Gargle

When you gargle, you will stimulate the vagus nerve, but as I tell you, do not overdo this activity, you can do a gargle session once a day.

Deep breathing

Deep breathing at the diaphragm level will tone your vagus nerve; oxygenation is key to reducing any stress process in the body.

Massages

Dare to give yourself the pleasure of a therapeutic massage a month, with someone with whom you feel comfortable, to help you relax the muscles of your face and your back. This helps a lot to keep the vagus nerve healthy.

Improve your posture

As I explain in this other article, improving your posture will align your vagus nerve, and that will immediately make it perform its functions correctly, hence practices like yoga help a lot.

Consume probiotics

The vagus nerve controls many of your stomach functions, so if you try to take care of your stomach, you will help your vagus nerve, the connection is bidirectional. It is scientifically proven that consuming probiotics will help you with that. In this other article, you find examples of probiotics along with my favorite foods to lower anxiety.

Socialize in trust

If you have a person in your life with whom you feel confident, go out more often with that person, talk to him on the phone, and try to connect with more. Positive socialization is key to this whole process. If you feel very disconnected from others, I share this article.

Respect the natural rhythms of your body

By this, I mean that if you are sleepy, you sleep... if you are hungry, eat... if you are thirsty, drink water ... And so, respect your body, listen to its needs and adapt your day to what your body is asking you what it needs.

I tell you some of the main points that your body needs to be in balance, check them, and share with us which one you will start.

When we lose the inner balance is that the existence of anxiety in our lives is facilitated, we should not pretend to remain in a static state always the same, that is not balance, balance is learning to move within your changes without getting too far from your center.

So now, I share some of the balance your body needs to be healthy and stop generating so much stress or anxiety.

Balance between being alert and relaxed

Your body needs you to be in a balance between moments of alertness and moments of relaxation, the moments of alertness being the least in your day. Alert is when you tense when you squeeze when you activate attitudes of apprehension, control, resistance, demand, and relaxation, it is when you are in the present, focused, and with your body relaxed.

Constant food

Your body needs that at least every 4 hours you give it some healthy food, which contains healthy calories, healthy fats, fiber, and nutrients as natural as possible.

Constant hydration

Of the same importance that food has, water has it; you need to be constantly hydrated, when you are thirsty, it is because your body is already stressed, and it sends you the signal that you need it, the idea is that you drink at least 2 liters of water a day but distributed.

Restful sleep

You need at least 4 hours of running sleep, the ideal is between 6 to 8 hours, depending on each person, but above all, that your sleep is of quality because sometimes we sleep but do not rest for issues such as sleep apnea, squeeze jaw, temperature changes, etc.

Aerobic exercise

Your body also needs aerobic exercise that leads you to sweat a little, sweating is one of the best ways to release toxins from stress, walking, swimming and doing yoga or chi kun are excellent exercises for this.

Balance between tension and relaxation

Muscularly you need to be relaxed; this can be done by stretching in the mornings, going to massages, entering hot tubs, through osteopathy, or muscle relaxation techniques. This allows your body to function better because the muscles are not generating tension.

Breathing - oxygenation

It is really important that you breathe effectively, with your stomach relaxed, bringing oxygen to your diaphragm or stomach, so that the oxygen that enters actually relaxes your body.

Needs covered

Your body needs you to listen to it in its needs and that, as far as possible, do not crush it for a long time, such as going to the bathroom, drinking water, eating, or resting before you feel that your body is going to ask for it.

Hours of work and concentration controlled

To be in balance, you also need to alternate your work hours or concentration with moments of healthy recreation, such as stopping to walk or drink water every hour, is more than 1 hour sitting doing the same activity exhausts your body and your mind.

Mental relaxation

Your mind is also part of your body, specifically your brain, and your brain can get tired from being over activated for a long time, that is why meditation is to the mind like exercise to the body, you just need to close your eyes and feel your breathing for at least 1 minute a day, with that, you will allow your brain to rest for a few moments.

Emotional release

In the same way, your emotions live in your body, that's where they feel, and that's where they have an influence on your body muscularly, that's why for your body to be in balance, you need to focus on having your emotions in balance (this we will continue seeing in the month of March).

There are many activities that can help you achieve all this together, such as artistic or manual activities, free dancing, writing, and the exercises already mentioned.

Don't try to change everything at once

If you feel that it is a lot to do, do not try to change everything from one moment to another, focus on going to include activities that you feel are more necessary for your body than others, and little by little, your body will respond and restore its inner balance. It is not about "stop doing this or that," but "start doing this that does me good."

Cover your physical needs and allow your body to do the rest

Once you cover your needs, that you are rested with relaxation and physical activation exercises, with your emotions off the hook ... then, leave your body the rest and allow it to recover its balance on its own, without pressing it, without hurrying it, just watch it how it achieves it while you are in charge of not leaving your balance ranges.

In conclusion

Making allies of our body is that we can give it what it needs to restore its balance by itself, and much of this will be achieved thanks to the functions of the vagus nerve, pay attention, and you will see its benefits.